Challenging OCD in Young People with ASD

in the same series

Challenge Your OCD!
A CBT Workbook for Young People with ASD
Amita Jassi
Illustrated by Lisa Jo Robinson
ISBN 978 1 78775 286 3
eISBN 978 1 78775 287 0

by the same author

OCD and Autism
A Clinician's Guide to Adapting CBT
Ailsa Russell, Amita Jassi and Kate Johnston
Illustrated by David Russell
ISBN 978 1 78592 379 1
eISBN 978 1 78450 728 2

Can I tell you about OCD?
A guide for friends, family and professionals
Amita Jassi
Illustrated by Sarah Hull
ISBN 978 1 84905 381 5
eISBN 978 0 85700 736 0

The Parents' Guide to Body Dysmorphic Disorder
How to Support Your Child, Teen or Young Adult
Nicole Schnackenberg, Benedetta Monzani and Amita Jassi
Foreword by Rob Willson and David Veale
ISBN 978 1 78775 113 2
eISBN 978 1 78775 114 9

Appearance Anxiety
A Guide to Understanding Body Dysmorphic Disorder for Young People, Families and Professionals
National and Specialist OCD, BDD and Related Disorders Service, Maudsley Hospital
ISBN 978 1 78592 456 9
eISBN 978 1 78450 832 6

CHALLENGING OCD IN YOUNG PEOPLE WITH ASD

A CBT Manual for Therapists

AMITA JASSI

Illustrated by Lisa Jo Robinson

Jessica Kingsley Publishers
London and Philadelphia

First published in Great Britain in 2021 by Jessica Kingsley Publishers
An Hachette Company

1

A CIP catalogue record for this title is available from the British Library and the Library of Congress

ISBN 978 1 78775 288 7
eISBN 978 1 78775 289 4

Printed and bound in Great Britain by CPI Group

Jessica Kingsley Publishers' policy is to use papers that are natural, renewable and recyclable products and made from wood grown in sustainable forests. The logging and manufacturing processes are expected to conform to the environmental regulations of the country of origin.

Jessica Kingsley Publishers
73 Collier Street
London N1 9BE, UK

www.jkp.com

Contents

Acknowledgements 9

INTRODUCTION 11

SESSION 1: INTRODUCTION AND LEARNING ABOUT OCD 17
SET AGENDA 17
LEARNING ABOUT CBT FOR OCD 18
GETTING TO KNOW YOU 18
WHAT IS OCD? 19
WHAT CAUSES OCD? 19
OCD IS NOT YOU! 20
HOMEWORK SESSION 1 21

SESSION 2: LEARNING ABOUT ASD AND OCD 23
SET AGENDA 23
RECAP: SESSION 1 23
HOMEWORK REVIEW 24
WHAT IS ASD? 24
DIFFERENCES BETWEEN OCD AND ASD 24
HOMEWORK SESSION 2 26

SESSION 3: LEARNING ABOUT ANXIETY 27
SET AGENDA 27
RECAP: SESSION 2 27
HOMEWORK REVIEW 27
WHAT IS ANXIETY? 28
WHY DO WE GET ANXIOUS? 28
ANXIETY RATING SCALE 30
HOMEWORK SESSION 3 31

SESSION 4: LEARNING ABOUT ANXIETY AND OCD 33
SET AGENDA 33
RECAP: SESSION 3 33
HOMEWORK REVIEW 33
ANXIETY HABITUATION 34
THE OCD CYCLE 35
WHAT HAPPENS TO ANXIETY IN OCD? 36
HOW TO BREAK THE OCD CYCLE 36
ANXIETY HABITUATION WHEN BREAKING THE OCD CYCLE 37
HOMEWORK SESSION 4 37

SESSION 5: SETTING UP A PLAN 39
SET AGENDA 39
RECAP: SESSION 4 39
HOMEWORK REVIEW 39
WHAT IS ERP? 40
OCD HIERARCHY 40
GOALS 41
HOMEWORK SESSION 5 41

SESSION 6: CHALLENGING OCD USING ERP 43
SET AGENDA 43
RECAP: SESSION 5 43
HOMEWORK REVIEW 43
CBT FOR OCD QUIZ! 44
FIRST ERP TASK! 44
HOMEWORK SESSION 6 48

SESSION 7: CHALLENGING OCD USING ERP (AND OCD REVIEW) 49
SET AGENDA 49
RECAP: SESSION 6 49
HOMEWORK REVIEW 49
REVIEW OCD 50
ERP TASK! 51
HOMEWORK SESSION 7 51

SESSION 8: CHALLENGING OCD USING ERP 53
SET AGENDA 53
RECAP: SESSION 7 53
HOMEWORK REVIEW 53
ERP TASK! 54
OCD STEPS 54
HOMEWORK SESSION 8 55

SESSION 9: CHALLENGING OCD USING ERP 57
- SET AGENDA 57
- RECAP: SESSION 8 57
- HOMEWORK REVIEW 57
- ERP TASK! 58
- THINGS TO HELP YOU DO ERP 58
- HOMEWORK SESSION 9 59

SESSION 10: CHALLENGING OCD USING ERP 61
- SET AGENDA 61
- RECAP: SESSION 9 61
- HOMEWORK REVIEW 61
- ERP TASK! 61
- HOMEWORK SESSION 10 62

SESSION 11: CHALLENGING OCD USING ERP 63
- SET AGENDA 63
- RECAP: SESSION 10 63
- HOMEWORK REVIEW 63
- ERP TASK! 64
- HOMEWORK SESSION 11 64

SESSION 12: CHALLENGING OCD USING ERP 65
- SET AGENDA 65
- RECAP: SESSION 11 65
- HOMEWORK REVIEW 65
- ERP TASK! 66
- RULES FOR CHALLENGING OCD 66
- HOMEWORK SESSION 12 66

SESSION 13: CHALLENGING OCD USING ERP 69
- SET AGENDA 69
- RECAP: SESSION 12 69
- HOMEWORK REVIEW 69
- ERP TASK! 69
- HOMEWORK SESSION 13 70

SESSION 14: CHALLENGING OCD USING ERP (AND OCD REVIEW) 71
- SET AGENDA 71
- RECAP: SESSION 13 71
- HOMEWORK REVIEW 71
- REVIEW OCD 72
- ERP TASK! 72
- HOMEWORK SESSION 14 73

SESSIONS 15–18: CHALLENGING OCD USING ERP – YOU TAKE CHARGE 75
SET AGENDA 75
RECAP: PREVIOUS SESSION 75
HOMEWORK REVIEW 75
ERP TASK! 76
THINGS TO HELP YOU DO ERP 76
HOMEWORK SESSIONS 15–18 77

SESSION 19: CHALLENGING OCD USING ERP AND GETTING READY FOR THE FINISH .. 79
SET AGENDA 79
RECAP: SESSION 18 79
HOMEWORK REVIEW 79
ERP OR EXTREME TASK! 80
GETTING READY FOR THE FINISH 80
HOMEWORK SESSION 19 80

SESSION 20: RELAPSE PREVENTION PLAN 81
SET AGENDA 81
RECAP: SESSION 19 81
HOMEWORK REVIEW 81
RELAPSE PREVENTION PLAN 82
REVIEW OCD 82
PLANNING AHEAD 83
CERTIFICATE 83

Appendix: Things to Help You in Treatment 85
DIFFERENT FEELINGS 85
LEARNING ABOUT THOUGHTS 85
HELPFUL THOUGHTS 87
ASK OTHERS TO CHALLENGE OCD 87
DO A SURVEY OR FIND OUT FACTS 88
MANAGING ASD-RELATED STRESS 89

Follow-Up 1–4: Review Progress and Plan 91
SET AGENDA 91
REVIEW AND PLAN 91
REVIEW AND MEASURE OCD 92
LOOKING TO THE FUTURE (FOLLOW-UP 4) 92

References 93

Acknowledgements

I would like to thank my colleagues (both past and present) at the National and Specialist OCD, BDD and Related Disorders Team for Young People, South London and Maudsley NHS Trust, UK. There are too many to mention but they have each contributed to the development of this treatment in different ways. In particular, I wish to thank Victoria Hallett, Gazal Jones, Zoe Kindynis, Benedetta Monzani, Lauren Peile and Kelly Wood for their helpful contributions. Thank you to Olivia Brooks-Wilkins who assisted with the illustration development of the OCD character used in this manual and the accompanying workbook.

I wish to acknowledge the two fantastic OCD treatment manuals available that have helped shape this one. These are *OCD and Autism: A Clinician's Guide to Adapting CBT* by Ailsa Russell, Amita Jassi and Kate Johnston and *OCD – Tools to Help Young People Fight Back! A CBT Manual for Therapists* by Cynthia Turner, Georgina Krebs and Chloe Volz (see References for details). Thank you to Georgina Krebs and Ailsa Russell for supporting the development and evaluation of this treatment for young people with ASD.

I wish to thank South London and Maudsley NHS Trust for the space and time to develop and trial this treatment, and the Biomedical Research Council for providing funding for the development of the accompanying workbook.

Finally, I wish to express my gratitude to all the young people and families I have had the privilege to work with over the years. This has given me incredible insight into their experiences, which has helped to develop this treatment. I hope it will benefit many more people out there.

Acknowledgements

INTRODUCTION

This therapist manual and accompanying workbook have been developed for the treatment of obsessive compulsive disorder (OCD) in young people with autism spectrum disorder (ASD). You will notice the term 'young people/person with ASD' is used throughout this therapist manual. However, recent feedback from people with ASD has suggested that some prefer identity-first language ('autistic young people/person') as opposed to person-first language ('young people/person with autism'). It is important when working with young people and their parents that you ask them what they prefer and if they prefer 'autism', 'ASD' or 'autism spectrum condition' ('ASC').

High rates of comorbidity between ASD and OCD are well established; a meta-analysis of 31 studies indicated that over 17 per cent of youth with ASD meet diagnostic criteria for OCD (Steensel, Bögels & Perrin, 2011). Cognitive behaviour therapy (CBT) has a robust evidence base and is recommended as the first-line treatment for young people with OCD (Geller & March, 2012; National Institute for Health and Clinical Excellence, 2005). A number of studies have directly compared CBT for OCD outcomes in young people with and without ASD, demonstrating that those with ASD have inferior outcomes at post-treatment (Murray *et al.*, 2015) and six month follow-up (Griffiths *et al.*, 2017). These findings highlight the need to individualize standard CBT protocols to better suit the developmental profile of young people with ASD.

Research exploring CBT for OCD in young people with ASD describes a wide-ranging set of CBT modifications (see Table I.1) and has found that it can be an effective treatment in young people with ASD when appropriately tailored to their developmental profile (Elliott & Fitzsimons, 2014; Farrell *et al.*, 2016; Krebs, Murray & Jassi, 2016; Lehmkuhl *et al.*, 2008; Nadeau *et al.*, 2013; Reaven & Hepburn, 2003; Rooney *et al.*, 2011; Russell *et al.*, 2013). Drawing on this research, this manual and accompanying workbook follow a CBT programme for OCD incorporating suggested modifications. The workbook and manual have been used with a group of young people and we have found better treatment outcomes compared to studies involving those who have received unmodified CBT (Jassi *et al.*, submitted). As well as a reduction in OCD severity, this treatment leads to a reduction in family accommodation and an increase in psychosocial functioning (Jassi *et al.*, submitted). There are typically three phases of treatment: education on OCD and anxiety, exposure and response prevention (ERP) and relapse prevention. This manual is written based on the assumption therapists using it have a working knowledge of both OCD and ASD and have some experience of delivering CBT with ERP.

This package of CBT for OCD for young people with ASD includes 20 weekly sessions, with four follow-up reviews, which are recommended to be completed at one, three, six and 12 months after the weekly sessions end. It is recommended the 20 weekly sessions are completed within a 25-week timeframe to ensure that there is the momentum needed for treatment to be effective. Evidence suggests extending treatment from 14 to 20 sessions for young people with ASD leads to further treatment gains, for example, there is a significant reduction in OCD severity in this treatment period (Jassi *et al.*, submitted). This CBT package is extended to accommodate modifications needed for young people with ASD, for example additional time for education on anxiety. The pace and content for each session has been based on clinical experience of what typically is covered; however, there will be variation across individuals, so you can use this as a guide and move through sessions more quickly or slowly based on your clinical judgement. There are optional modules ('Things to help you in treatment') in the Appendix at the end of the workbook and described in this manual, which can be added in where appropriate, so this may impact on the pacing of sessions. Typically, we recommend up to six sessions on the education phase as you may need to add modules including 'Different feelings' and 'Learning about thoughts' for young people with ASD.

The treatment package has primarily been used with young people aged 11 years and above and for those without a learning disability (full-scale IQ > 70). Young people with ASD may have specific learning difficulties such as dyslexia. This treatment is appropriate for them, with relevant adaptations made based on clinical judgement, for example less reliance on written materials.

Throughout this manual, the term 'young person' is used to refer to both children and adolescents, and the term 'parent' is used to refer to the child's biological parent, step-parent, carer or guardian. Ideally, parents and family members who are involved in the OCD or reside with the young person should be present for the therapy. However, given the practicalities and time commitment needed, we recommend that at least one parent or family member attends the sessions. For some young people, it is helpful to have the parent or family member in for the entire session, and for others, it may be helpful to ask them to join at the end of the session to get feedback and highlight what they can do to help with homework tasks. It may be helpful to record the sessions for family members who are unable to attend. Recordings can also be useful for the young person to listen to in order to remind them of the content of sessions and to strengthen and promote generalization of their learning.

It is helpful to make sure from the outset that the family understand their important role in treatment. For example, we know all families accommodate OCD, therefore it is helpful if they attend and understand the education phase of treatment and appreciate the principles of ERP. This will help them when they are reducing their accommodation of OCD, as well as supporting the young person with their homework tasks. As treatment progresses, we encourage the young person and parent to take more of a lead in sessions, building up their confidence in challenging OCD. This supports them to become their own therapists, in preparation for when regular sessions end. This manual is written assuming the parent is in the session; if they are not, arrange to feed back the main points at the end of the session. It is helpful to encourage the young person to give the feedback, so you can check their understanding.

The manual walks you through the accompanying workbook, by explaining the content of each session. This is primarily to assist therapists to gain experience and confidence in treating OCD in young people with ASD, considering the adaptations needed. For experienced therapists, the manual simply highlights the topic to be discussed with the young person and parent, and the therapist should feel comfortable to hold a discussion with the child using their own language and examples. While the body of the manual incorporates modifications for young people with ASD, some important considerations are highlighted as a 'therapist note'. Each session can be set up to last for around 60 minutes; however, some young people may need slightly shorter or longer sessions. Some may not tolerate the longer sessions as they may struggle with the interpersonal demands of the session as well as the CBT content. Others may need more time to absorb the information from sessions or require a break halfway through. It is important to be aware of this and tailor session length to suit the individual. If a young person wants to take up session time talking about their special interests or other topics, you can consider allowing time at the end to do this, as a reward for completing the session.

While this manual will discuss each session in turn, it is important to hold in mind broader modifications to CBT needed for many young people with ASD. These have been incorporated into the workbook as much as possible and are summarized in Table I.1 (taken from Krebs, Murray & Jassi, 2016) for you to hold in mind to further adapt treatment:

Table I.1: Modifications to CBT to accommodate ASD profiles

	Modification to standard CBT	Reason for modification
Format of CBT	Greater use of visual materials and worksheets	Language and/or communication difficulties
	Simplify language and concepts	Difficulties in understanding information
	Greater repetition of key psychological concepts	Processing speed and/or working memory impairments
	Short breaks throughout sessions, particularly psychoeducation sessions	Impairments in attention, processing speed or working memory
	Sessions highly structured with agenda and timings explicitly shared	Need for routine and predictability Executive functioning difficulties
	Directive, explicit and factual style of therapy	Literal communication style
	Rules for conversations, e.g. turn taking, interrupting, etc.	Difficulties in reading social situations
	'Download time' at end of every session to discuss special interests	To reduce tangential conversations during the session and reward at the end of the session
Content of CBT	Extended psychoeducation about anxiety, e.g. education on different emotions, where anxiety presents in the body	Poor emotional recognition and understanding Attention difficulties Difficulty understanding information
	Use of the young person's idiosyncratic words/phrases	Communication difficulties
	Use of traffic light system to rate anxiety Focus on a specific symptom (e.g. heart rate) to facilitate rating anxiety	Difficulties seeing emotions on continuous scale Poor emotional understanding and communication
	Hierarchies developed around specific goals	Concrete thinking style Limited motivation
	Smaller steps in ERP tasks	Distress intolerance
	Taking photos and videos of ERP tasks	Difficulty generalizing Concrete thinking style
	Increased involvement of parents, i.e. leading ERP tasks in sessions	Difficulty generalizing
	Regular home-based ERP sessions	Difficulty generalizing
	Working with school and other systems	Difficulty generalizing Need to optimize functioning in all domains by ensuring appropriate support in place for neurodevelopmental needs
	Parents/therapist modelling tasks	Difficulties in carrying out task with instructions only

Before starting treatment, it is assumed the young person has been assessed to have diagnoses of OCD and ASD. As part of this assessment, it is recommended that a validated measure of OCD is completed and that this is repeated at review points, as detailed in this manual, to track progress in treatment. The recommended clinician-administered measure is the Children's Yale Brown Obsessive Compulsive Scale (CY-BOCS) (Scahill *et al.*, 1997). An alternative, if time is limited, is a questionnaire called the Children's Obsessional Compulsive Inventory-Revised (ChOCI-R) (Shafran *et al.*, 2003), which comes in a young person and a parent version. These measures record the same information for obsessions and compulsions: time, interference, distress, resistance and control. Ideally, both the clinician and self-report measures should be completed to get an overview of OCD from different perspectives.

This therapist manual and CBT workbook have been developed in a clinical service with feedback from young people, families and therapists. To enable this treatment to continue to improve outcomes for young people with OCD and ASD, we would be grateful for feedback from young people, families and therapists using the workbook and manual outside our clinical setting. Please email the author (Amita Jassi) on ocdbdd.camhs@slam.nhs.uk if you wish to provide feedback.

Finally, you will notice icons in the workbook; they mean the following:

The pencil icon means the young person has to write something in their workbook.

The download icon means that page is downloadable if the young person needs additional copies or copies are needed outside the workbook for practical reasons, for example if parents need to complete a sheet in parallel to the young person and they only have one workbook between them. Pages marked with this symbol can be downloaded from https://library.jkp.com/redeem using the code FAUHONE.

Session 1

INTRODUCTION AND LEARNING ABOUT OCD

SESSION 1 PLAN

- Set agenda
- Learning about CBT for OCD
- Getting to know you
- What is OCD?
- What causes OCD?
- OCD is not you!
- Set homework

SET AGENDA

Explain to the young person and parent that at the beginning of every session up to ten minutes will be spent setting up a plan for the session. Open the workbook at Session 1 to show them what will be included today and ask them if there is anything they would like to add to the session plan. Young people with ASD may value having rules for sessions and may need the time structured for them to allow the session content to be covered. You may wish to mention at this stage that for treatment to work, it is important to ensure that all the sections are covered, so you may need to move things on. You can show the young person that they can tick off points on an agenda, and if helpful, times can be put next to each point to make sure everything is covered.

You can ask the young person and family how they feel about an hour session; ask them if they think they will be able to concentrate, whether they will need a break and so on. If they are unsure, you can suggest you see how today goes and then review at the end when planning next week's session if they needed a break. As a therapist, you will get a sense as the session progresses about whether they have been able to concentrate and take in all the information, so you can tailor the next session accordingly.

You should encourage the parent to remain for the entire session, and for them to do this at least for the entire education phase if possible (the first six sessions). You can explain it is important that everyone understands OCD and how to challenge it in the same way, as this will give them the best chance of treatment working. If the young person does not want their parent in the room, you can explore the reasons for this and see if these can be resolved. If they cannot, a parent check-in at the end of the session to give feedback is important and should be added to the agenda.

To summarize what they will do in today's session, explain that you will be using some time to get to know the young person and learn about OCD.

LEARNING ABOUT CBT FOR OCD

Introduce the workbook to the young person and parent and share with them the outline of what sessions involve. Explain what CBT stands for and highlight that they will be offered up to 20 sessions of CBT and, ideally, they should have a session every week. The goal is to complete sessions within 25 weeks to allow for holidays or if you or they are unwell. Explain it is important to have sessions within this timeframe to keep the momentum of treatment as we know this is important when challenging OCD. Some young people with ASD like to have appointments set out in advance to make things predictable. It is helpful to have them set on the same day and time if possible, to establish a routine.

Talk the young person and parent through the overview of what treatment involves, as set out in the workbook. When discussing the CBT programme, it is important to highlight the review points, so they are aware that progress will be tracked. Homework tasks in between sessions should also be mentioned, and emphasize that these are just as important as the weekly meetings (if not more so). Explain that daily practice is vital in getting better from OCD, allowing them to apply what they have learned in session to their 'real life' at home. Practising once a week is not enough.

Explain to the young person and parent that CBT for OCD involves you all working together to challenge OCD step by step. It works best if the plan is followed as set out in the workbook. It is helpful to highlight that CBT involves training them up on the skills they need to challenge OCD in the longer term. As treatment progresses, they will take the lead more often, giving them the confidence to keep challenging OCD when sessions end.

GETTING TO KNOW YOU

The therapist should spend some time at the start of the session getting to know the young person. This allows you to get information about what the young person's wider life looks like outside their OCD, including their special interests, which can be creatively incorporated into their treatment. This part of the session can be used to get a sense of how the young person communicates, their social interaction and how they manage with the pacing of sessions. You can explicitly ask them about how they prefer to communicate and what helps them to learn.

WHAT IS OCD?

Ask the young person and parent what they know about OCD and explore their existing knowledge. If they have not already covered this, explain that OCD stands for obsessive compulsive disorder. Define obsessions as unwanted thoughts, worries, pictures, urges or doubts that pop into people's heads and that typically make someone feel anxious, uncomfortable or upset. Define compulsions as the actions or behaviours young people with OCD do to make the obsession go away or to reduce anxiety or discomfort. Sometimes it just doesn't feel 'right' until they have done the compulsion in a certain way. It is helpful to highlight at this stage that some compulsions are visible to other people (e.g. hand washing, organizing, tapping), while others are done inside the head (e.g. counting, praying). Other people in the family may also find they have to do compulsions for OCD (e.g. extra laundry, giving reassurance).

Explain that while most people have obsessions and compulsions, the reason we call it a disorder is because the obsessions and compulsions are annoying, distressing and get in the way of what we really want to be doing. It is helpful to share that OCD is very common and that one or two in every 100 young people have it. If they are at school or college, you can ask them how many young people attend and then give them a concrete number of how many will have OCD. If they do not attend school or college, you can use other examples: on a bus there are often a hundred passengers, so one or two of them could have OCD.

To support the young person to link this information to their OCD, invite them to look at the examples in the workbook and to tick the obsessions and compulsions that relate to them. If their symptoms are not on the list, there is space for them to add their own examples. If they are struggling, it can be helpful to ask their parents what they think. You can link back to the 'Getting to know you' section and ask if the obsessions and compulsions affect any of the areas they discussed and, if so, in what way. This can help them to think about the 'disorder' part of OCD.

WHAT CAUSES OCD?

You may find it helpful to start by asking the young person and parent what they think is the cause of OCD. This can elicit their beliefs about OCD, which are helpful to address in treatment. For example, parents may believe that the OCD is their fault in some way, owing to their genes or parenting style. Alternatively, the parent may blame the young person, thinking it's a behavioural difficulty under their control.

Once you have heard from the young person and parent, it is important to challenge any unhelpful beliefs, for example emphasize that OCD is not the young person being disobedient. The most important thing to share is that it is nobody's fault the young person has OCD. It can be helpful to relate this to examples of other illnesses that people get that are not their fault but require management and treatment to get better, such as cancer and diabetes.

Share with the family that no one knows the cause of OCD, but research has shown that there may be several different contributing factors. These include:

- having low levels of serotonin in the brain (hence why Selective Serotonin Reuptake Inhibitors or SSRI medication is prescribed)
- having a family or genetic 'risk', as often we hear other family members have OCD or other related difficulties
- having experienced stressful events in the past that may relate to OCD
- being someone who generally gets anxious about things.

It is important to share that none of these factors alone is thought to cause OCD; for example, if it was all about low levels of serotonin then medication would work completely. It is likely to be a combination of these and other factors. You should explain that not knowing the cause for OCD is actually not that important as we know CBT can work regardless. It works for different types of OCD, for people from varied backgrounds and with different experiences. You can use the following analogy if helpful: if they had broken their leg, the doctor does not need to know how it happened to be able to treat it, as the treatment is the same regardless of how it happened.

OCD IS NOT YOU!

In treatment, a helpful technique is to externalize OCD from the young person. This technique is taken from narrative therapy, and Dr John March incorporated this into OCD treatment for young people (see March & Mulle, 1998). This process encourages the young person and family to see OCD as separate from the young person and something that can be challenged together. This helps the young person to build insight that these thoughts and behaviours are different from other types of thoughts and behaviours, and it reinforces the idea in families that this is not something the young person is doing on purpose.

In this section of the workbook, different ideas for how to support the young person and parent to externalize OCD are suggested, such as drawing the OCD, naming it or writing words to describe it. Some young people with ASD may enjoy the creativity involved in externalizing OCD in this way, whereas others may have a more literal thinking style and prefer to call it OCD. It is best to give the young person the choice and follow their lead. Throughout treatment, it is important to use the language, 'What is OCD making you do?' (if the young person has named their OCD, replace 'OCD' with the given name when speaking about it).

HOMEWORK SESSION 1

When summarizing what CBT involves at the beginning of the session you will have spoken about the importance of homework. You may wish to emphasize the importance of this again here. For young people with ASD, you may need to set out a plan with them for when they will complete their homework before the next session. Ask them if there is anything else they need to help them complete homework, for example parents reminding them.

In order for the young person and their parents to consolidate their learning from the session, ask them to read over Session 1 in their workbook. While doing so, ask them to write three things they learned during the session and any questions they have over the week. You will see there is space to add extra homework if you feel this is needed. This can include finishing sections of Session 1 if they were not completed and if they are appropriate to be completed independently.

To further their understanding of OCD, you can ask the young person and their families to watch the following:

- www.ocdisnotme.com – a short film of young people and their parents sharing their experience of living with OCD and their journey through CBT for OCD, including in some cases using this manual and workbook.
- http://cargocollective.com/salvadormaldonado/over-and-over-and-over-again – a short animation of a young person sharing his experience of OCD.

There may be other websites or videos you are aware of that could be helpful to share at this stage.

Session 2

LEARNING ABOUT ASD AND OCD

SESSION 2 PLAN

- Set agenda
- Recap of Session 1
- Homework review
- What is ASD?
- Differences between OCD and ASD
- Set homework

SET AGENDA

Refer to the workbook and explain to the young person and parent what will be included in the session today. Give them an opportunity to add anything to the agenda that they feel is relevant. If helpful, you can add timings to each section to ensure everything is covered, and that there is a break and parent check-in time if they are not in the session. This process of agenda setting will be the same for every session, so will not be repeated moving forward through the manual.

To summarize what will be included in today's session, you can share that you will be focusing on learning more about ASD and thinking about the differences between OCD and ASD.

RECAP: SESSION 1

Spend some time with the young person and parent to review what was covered in Session 1 to ensure they have understood the contents before moving on today.

HOMEWORK REVIEW

Following on from reviewing the last session, look over the three things they learned from Session 1 and any questions they have. You can ask them what they thought about the videos and what they learned from watching them. Review any additional homework you set.

If they did not complete their homework, it is important to spend some time thinking with the young person about possible reasons for this and to consider together some possible solutions. Ideas may include setting an alarm on their phone as a reminder, drawing out a visual timetable for homework tasks, or rewards from family if they complete homework.

WHAT IS ASD?

Before beginning this section, ask the young person and parent about their understanding of ASD and what support they have had related to the diagnosis. It is helpful to get an idea of their existing knowledge, so that you are not repeating information. You may need to provide more detailed information if they have not received ASD support in the past.

Explain that the reason this is being covered in the session is because you will be thinking about the differences between ASD and OCD and some of the overlaps, as it can sometimes get confusing. Share with them that it is important to be clear on what is OCD and not ASD as this treatment focuses on challenging OCD.

Explain that ASD stands for autism spectrum disorder and is a short-hand way of describing a group of people who have a particular personality style or some differences in the ways their brain and bodies work. ASD in particular impacts on social interaction, communication, interests and behaviours. This is something people are born with and not something that we are trying to 'cure' or 'fix'. Like OCD, there have been possible causes for ASD explored, including genetics and having ASD traits in families, but it is not clear what the cause of ASD is. ASD is very common as around one in 100 people have it.

Invite the young person to look at this section in their workbook, to review the list and tick characteristics that they feel apply to them. They can add information in the space given within each box. If they struggle to do this or do not have insight into their difficulties, you can invite their parents to help. This section will give you further insight into the young person's ASD and can help you to think about what modifications you may need to incorporate into your sessions.

DIFFERENCES BETWEEN OCD AND ASD

A key purpose of this session is to support the young person and parent to think about the differences between ASD and OCD. This section of the workbook highlights some of the differences between the two conditions.

Refer to the two circles on the Venn diagram and explain that they each represent OCD and ASD respectively. Starting with obsessions, ask the young person and parent what obsessions refer to OCD, as discussed in the last session. Using concrete examples of the obsessions they shared in Session 1, remind them that these are thoughts, worries, images, doubts and urges that pop up and are unwanted (i.e. ego-dystonic). Explain that it can be confusing as in ASD the word 'obsession' is used differently. Again, you can ask them what they think or explain that this can refer to special interests that are enjoyable to think about (i.e. ego-syntonic). It would be useful to use the concrete examples that they just shared in the 'What is ASD?' section. Here it is important to highlight that, in OCD, obsessions are unpleasant and unwanted and cause distress, whereas in ASD, they tend to be pleasant, wanted and enjoyable. There is also a difference in how obsessions are experienced: they pop in and out in OCD, but in ASD they are more focused and something to think about intensely.

THERAPIST NOTE

Often young people with ASD struggle to understand how thoughts work or the different types of thoughts they may experience. This may become evident when doing the section on obsessions. If they are struggling, they may find it helpful to do the optional module 'Learning about thoughts' (see the Appendix in the workbook and in this manual for guidance). You can do this module at other times if it is clear that the young person would benefit from a better understanding of their mental world. Another reason to do this module is if you think it is helpful for them to know that people without OCD get similar thoughts, albeit that they do not cause distress or lead to compulsions or avoidance.

Moving on to behaviours, ask the young person and parent to think about how these differ between OCD and ASD. You should highlight that, in OCD, behaviours are called compulsions that are performed to try and reduce anxiety or uncomfortable feelings or to stop something bad from happening. You can use their examples from Session 1 to relate to this. It is important to share that in OCD these behaviours are really annoying and distressing. People do not want to do the behaviours and, if they were less scared or worried, would not need to do them. If possible, try to give concrete examples of behaviours in ASD that might be similar to those in OCD (e.g. lining things up, following a specific routine), explaining that these may not have a set purpose like they do in OCD. Such ASD behaviours are typically not distressing and at times can be enjoyable. At this point, you can ask the young person and parent to add anything into the two circles that they feel would be relevant to this discussion.

THERAPIST NOTE

In attempting to disentangle ASD repetitive behaviours and OCD compulsions, you can consider the onset and course of the behaviours. A 'new' phenomenon with an onset in late childhood or adolescence is more likely to be part of OCD. Repetitive behaviours are likely to have been around since early childhood.

When discussing the differences between ASD and OCD behaviours, there may be some behaviours where it is unclear if they are completely ego-syntonic or ego-dystonic. However, if it is causing distress or disruption to the young person's functioning, it can be useful to consider it as a behavour to target in treatment.

HOMEWORK SESSION 2

In order for the young person and their parents to consolidate their learning from the session, ask them to read over Session 2 for homework. While doing so, ask them to write three things they learned during the session and any questions they have over the week. There is space to add extra homework if you feel this is needed, for example finishing sections of Session 2 if they were not completed.

Invite the young person and family to add information to the 'What is ASD?' section in the workbook. This may be things they already know, or you can ask them to go away and have a look at some information, such as the National Autistic Society's website. To further their understanding of ASD, you can ask the young person and their family to watch the following:

- www.youtube.com/watch?v=6fy7gUIp8Ms – a short animation explaining what autism is.

There may be other websites or videos you are aware of that may be helpful to share at this stage. If there were any issues with completing homework last week, revisit the ideas discussed at the beginning of the session to ensure they have a concrete and specific plan for completion.

Session 3

LEARNING ABOUT ANXIETY

SESSION 2 PLAN

- Set agenda
- Recap of Session 2
- Homework review
- What is anxiety?
- Why do we get anxious?
- Anxiety rating scale
- Set homework

SET AGENDA

Refer to the workbook and explain to the young person and parent what will be included in this session. Explain that today the focus will be on learning about anxiety as this is a feeling that is part of OCD, and in order to challenge OCD, they need to know how anxiety works.

RECAP: SESSION 2

Spend some time with the young person and parent to review what was covered in Session 2 and to ensure that they have understood the contents before moving on.

HOMEWORK REVIEW

Following on from reviewing the last session, you can review the three things they learned from Session 2 and if they had any questions. You can ask them about any new information they found when researching ASD, what they thought of the video, and how they think this relates to them. Review whether they have done any additional homework you set, such as completing unfinished sections from Session 2. Again, if they did not complete homework in this or any future sessions, discuss possible reasons and solutions for this.

WHAT IS ANXIETY?

Before you start this section, ask the young person and parent what they think anxiety is and add information to this if they are struggling. Explain that it is very important to understand how anxiety feels and why we have it, to help us challenge OCD. You can introduce the idea that OCD uses anxiety to make the young person do what OCD wants.

Explain that anxiety is a normal feeling that everyone experiences. If the parent is there, you can ask them to share if they get anxious, share with them that you get anxious and, if they have a pet, you can explain that they get anxious too! You can all share what makes each of you anxious and encourage the young person to think of examples outside OCD. This process, and giving concrete examples, will normalize the fact that everyone gets anxious. It is important for parents to recognize their own anxiety and share this early on, as this can help them to relate to their child's OCD-related anxiety.

Referring to this section of the workbook, explain that anxiety involves physical sensations that happen in our body. Ask them to review the different physical sensations and tick which sensations apply to them. To support them to do this, you can use one of the examples they shared of what makes them anxious and ask them to think back to that situation and what they noticed changed in their body. If they are struggling, you can give your examples or ask their parent to share what physical sensations they experience. If they are able to complete this exercise, they can add additional sensations that may not be included on the list.

The key in this exercise is to ensure that the young person is focusing on physical sensations of anxiety rather than their thoughts. This is to help them with the next section when you discuss the fight or flight response. If, through this exercise, you notice they are struggling to disentangle anxiety from other emotions, you can refer to the Appendix in the workbook and in this manual to support the young person with emotional literacy ('Different feelings' section).

THERAPIST NOTE

Many young people with ASD struggle to identify physical changes in their body. If they are unable to do this, it is still important to cover the following sections in Session 3. For young people who cannot recognize symptoms of anxiety, it may be helpful to consider alternative external means of measuring this when you start to rate anxiety later in the session, for example wearable devices that measure heart rate.

WHY DO WE GET ANXIOUS?

Explain that when the brain registers there is a danger or threat, a chemical called adrenaline is released and physical changes in our body happen automatically. This is called the 'fight or flight response'. At this time, our body helps us to stand up and fight the danger or to run away and take flight. Linking back to the previous section, explain that the physical sensations listed happen for a variety of reasons, including:

- Sweating – to cool the body down to prevent it overheating when in fight or flight.
- Feeling sick/butterflies/wobbly feeling in stomach – movement of blood away from the gut to muscles in legs and arms.
- Headache – constriction of blood vessels in some body parts.
- Dry mouth – inhibition of salivation.
- Shaky arms/legs – muscles tense and primed for action.
- Heart racing/fast breathing – acceleration of heart/lungs to pump oxygen to muscles.

It is helpful to explain to young people and parents that anxiety, and these physical changes in the body, are not dangerous and do not cause damage.

It is important to share that the fight or flight response is a very old, evolutionary system, which has developed in humans over thousands of years. It may be helpful to explain that it dates back to our cave-dwelling times, when there were very frequent and 'real' threats to human life (e.g. sabre-tooth tigers!). The fight or flight response was essential to the human race surviving. However, as humankind has evolved, the system has not been updated and so sometimes the fight or flight response can get triggered when there is no 'real' danger to life. Invite them to think with you and their parents of situations where the fight or flight response can be helpful (e.g. if a car came speeding towards them) and times when it might be unhelpful (e.g. when you are giving a presentation). Ask them to write these examples down in the workbook. Highlight that in one situation there is actual threat to life and in the other there is not. Explain that thoughts in themselves can trigger anxiety, for example the thought of giving a presentation can make us feel nauseous. This is important in OCD, as obsessions are thoughts that trigger anxiety.

THERAPIST NOTE

Look out for any unhelpful beliefs the young person and parent may hold about anxiety. Young people with ASD tend to be black and white in their thinking and they may also struggle to understand what physical changes in their body mean – for example, 'My heart racing means I am having a heart attack, so it is dangerous.' It is important that these beliefs are challenged either through the education phase or while in the ERP phase, as this could potentially interfere in treatment. It may be helpful to explain in detail the physical changes in the body that happen when they are anxious and the reason for them, as described above. They can also test out their beliefs about anxiety – for example, that anxiety will get higher and higher and never come down – during the ERP phase of treatment.

ANXIETY RATING SCALE

Start this section by explaining that anxiety can be experienced at different levels; some things cause us to feel more anxious than others. Even though sometimes they can experience anxiety as really high, there may be things that do not make them anxious and things that may fall somewhere in between.

Explain to the young person that in order to overcome OCD, it is important not only to understand anxiety but also to have a way to communicate how anxious they feel. One way to do this is by developing a rating scale for anxiety to help them communicate how anxious they feel in different situations. Share the examples included in the workbook. Ask them whether they have used similar scales before and what has been helpful and unhelpful.

THERAPIST NOTE

Some young people with ASD struggle to put numbers to feelings, so you could try to use different colours or a traffic light system to help them to convey how they feel. Another way to support them to develop a system that works for them is to incorporate their special interests, for example different Doctor Who characters, with The Doctor representing low anxiety and a Dalek being the highest anxiety. Some young people with ASD struggle with having too many options of ratings within their scale, whether it is colours, numbers or their special interests, so you may wish to consider limiting their options and, say, just having three colours on their scale.

Once the type of scale has been decided on and the ratings have been identified (i.e. numbers, colours, special interests), invite the young person to draw their scale in the workbook, or download the traffic lights or thermometer scale if they have chosen one of them. Following this, ask them to think about different situations that make them experience different levels of anxiety and ensure that these are examples outside their OCD. Explain that this is important as this scale will be used like a ruler against which OCD will be measured. Additionally, by the end of treatment the hope is that OCD obsessions will trigger less anxiety, so it is important that the scale has anchor points that are more likely to remain consistent during therapy. For you as a therapist, this is really important as, if the young person over- or under-reports anxiety in relation to OCD, you have concrete examples to compare to.

It is often helpful to think about the two extreme ends first: a situation that makes them feel really relaxed (perhaps relating to their special interests) and a situation that would make them feel the most extreme anxiety they could imagine. Share with them that the latter is often a life-threatening situation that may not have happened, such as being surrounded by sharks in the sea. You can use examples they have shared with you so far in treatment (e.g. in the 'What is anxiety?' section) to complete anchors on the scale. It is unlikely that you will get this all completed in the session and they will need to finish this for homework, so prioritize getting an example for the top, middle and bottom of the scale.

When getting ratings for different situations for their scale, hook into the physical sensations they have shared with you in their workbook; for example, 'Think of a situation when your heart rate was so steady and normal that you did not even notice it. Now think of an example where your heart was beating really fast.'

In order to support the young person to complete their scale, you and their parent can share examples of what would make you relaxed, extremely anxious and somewhere in the middle. Ask the parents to support the young person to come up with examples based on what they have observed by asking them what situations make them anxious, how high they think this is and how they know this or what they notice, for example the young person is tense, pacing around or shouting.

THERAPIST NOTE

Anxiety responses often look different in the ASD population – they may exhibit more repetitive behaviours, verbal aggression, pacing, becoming clingy or struggle to separate and so on. It can be helpful to add these responses on the anxiety rating scale along with other physical anxiety sensations they experience, to further help to anchor the scale; for example, amber on the traffic light means tense muscles, voice getting louder, hands shaking.

HOMEWORK SESSION 3

A standard part of homework each week is for the young person and their parents to consolidate their learning by reading over the session in their workbook. While they are doing so, ask them to write three things they learned during the session and any questions they have over the week. You will see there is space to add homework if you feel this is needed; this can include finishing sections of Session 3 if they were not completed. Given that this is a standard part of homework, it will not be repeated in the manual going forward.

It is important for young people with ASD to use the time between Sessions 3 and 4 to notice physical symptoms of anxiety and tick them off or add them to the list in the workbook. They are likely to find this easier when in the moment, and parents can be helpful in this process by noticing when the young person is anxious and asking them to notice what is happening in their body.

As the young person is being asked to notice anxiety, ask them to rate their anxiety at the time so they get to practise using their rating scale and to complete their rating scale if this has not been done in the session.

In the workbook, ask the young person to keep a diary of their OCD between this and the next session and ask their family to do the same. They will see on the table to write down the date, what OCD made them do, made others do or made them avoid, and to note down how long they did this for or how many times. For the diary logging what others do for OCD, it is important to flag that this should include people outside the family, such as teachers at school and friends. Encourage them to try to complete the diary at least once a day. Explain that this is going to be valuable information for upcoming sessions.

Session 4

LEARNING ABOUT ANXIETY AND OCD

SESSION 4 PLAN

- Set agenda
- Recap of Session 3
- Homework review
- Anxiety habituation
- The OCD cycle
- What happens to anxiety in OCD?
- How to break the OCD cycle
- Anxiety habituation when breaking the OCD cycle
- Set homework

SET AGENDA

Refer to the workbook and explain to the young person and parent what will be included in the session today. Explain that they will learn more about anxiety and how this links to OCD, which is fundamental to developing a plan to challenge OCD.

RECAP: SESSION 3

Spend some time with the young person and parent to review what was covered in Session 3 and to ensure that they have understood the contents before moving on today.

HOMEWORK REVIEW

Review three things they learned from Session 3 and if they had any questions from the session. Review their anxiety symptoms and rating scale and ask how they found doing this. This will give you an idea of how easy or difficult this was for them. If it was difficult, you may wish to consider asking them to keep practising this week; if it was impossible for them to do, consider other options of measuring anxiety, such as wearable heart-rate devices. Spend a few minutes looking over their diaries and explain that you will come back to these later in the session. Check that they have done any additional homework you set, such as completing unfinished sections from Session 3. Again, if they did not complete homework in this or any future sessions, discuss possible reasons and solutions for this.

ANXIETY HABITUATION

Explain that in today's session they are going to learn more about anxiety and how it works. Ask if they have heard about anxiety habituation or if they know what it means. If they have not heard about it, explain that this describes what happens to anxiety over time when you face something scary and you do not do anything to bring anxiety down. Ask the young person to pick one of the examples from their anxiety rating scale from Session 3 or another non-OCD example of where they remained in the situation even though they felt anxious. It is helpful for them to choose an example of a situation they faced more than once.

Talk them through the anxiety diagram in the workbook, using their example. Support them to think back to the specific situation, asking them where they were, who they were with and anything else they remember. Ask them to think about their anxiety as they approached the situation, perhaps focusing on one specific anxiety physical sensation, such as their breathing. They would have noticed that at first their anxiety increased as they approached the situation (anticipatory anxiety) or when they were first in the situation. Ask them to think about what happened to their anxiety when they stayed in the situation; they would have experienced their anxiety peak and then potentially plateau or start to reduce. It is important to highlight that their anxiety eventually reduced without them having to do anything to bring it down. Ask their parent to share something that they had to face that made them anxious and explore the same process of habituation for them. This can help the young person understand that this process of habituation happens regardless of the fear and is something we all experience. Asking parents to share their experience of anxiety habituation as well as hearing their child's example can be a good way to address any unhelpful beliefs they may hold about what they should do when their child is anxious, for example remove the child from the situation.

Turn to the next anxiety diagram. Hopefully you have chosen an example of something the young person faced on more than one occasion, to illustrate what happens to anxiety when you face the same situation repeatedly. Ask them to talk through what happened to their anxiety the second time they faced the fear. Support them to share that the second time their anxiety would have risen, but not as high as the first time. Explain the process for the third time they faced a fear, that this time it would not have risen as much as the second time. Ask them what they think would happen the more they faced the same fear over and over again. They should be able to recognize that their anxiety would reduce each time and eventually the situation would not make them anxious. Again, invite parents to share their experiences of this process.

> **THERAPIST NOTE**
>
> It is important to explain to a young person with ASD that the anxiety curve shown in the workbook may not always be smooth; it may be slightly wavy, still lowering, but it may not just reduce in a linear manner. It is important to explain that in the diagram, with repeated exposure, even though there are three lines, it does not mean it only takes three times for anxiety to reduce – this is just to make the point that it gets easier each time. Additionally, it may be helpful to explain that we would not expect their anxiety to reduce beyond their initial anxiety (before they started the task) or to go to zero. This is to ensure they have realistic expectations of what will happen.

THE OCD CYCLE

Share with the young person and parent that they are going to now learn about how OCD works and the role of anxiety in the 'OCD cycle'. Ask them to turn to this section of the workbook and talk them through the diagram. Explain that this is an example of someone with OCD that involves checking the front door repeatedly. For this young person, the trigger of their obsession is leaving the house and the person has the obsession that the door is unlocked, and someone will come into their home. This makes them feel anxious and leads them to do a compulsion which involves them checking the door over and over again. This makes their anxiety go down temporarily, until the next time they leave the house. This then reinforces the obsession and makes the cycle go around and around and OCD gets stronger and makes the young person do more and more (or lengthier) compulsions.

> **THERAPIST NOTE**
>
> If you notice that the young person is struggling to disentangle thoughts, feelings and behaviours when completing the cycle, it is important to spend some time to support them before you continue with next sections of the treatment. Materials developed by Dr Paul Stallard can be helpful in supporting them with this (https://blogs.sch.gr/fmarvel/files/2014/04/Paul_Stallard_Think_Good_-_Feel_Good_.pdf).

Check they have understood the OCD cycle before moving on. Ask them to refer to the OCD diaries they completed for homework (Session 3 in the workbook) and choose one compulsion OCD made them do over the week. Turning to this section of the workbook, ask them to complete the OCD cycle using their example. Ask them specific questions about where they were at the time, so they refer to a concrete example for this exercise. Ask them to fill in the boxes accordingly. At this stage, it is important to emphasize that the OCD cycle is the same regardless of the young person's specific obsessions and compulsions. This includes what others have to do for OCD, as it is just someone else doing the compulsion instead of the young person. If you are aware the young person avoids things because of their OCD, you may wish to take the opportunity to share that avoidance is a way to stop this cycle starting by not facing the triggers, but this also keeps OCD going.

WHAT HAPPENS TO ANXIETY IN OCD?

Ask the young person what happens to anxiety in the OCD cycle. They should recognize that anxiety reduces when they do a compulsion, but that this is temporary until the next time OCD gets triggered. Share with the young person that it is not surprising OCD gets power, as it gives you a way to bring those uncomfortable feelings of anxiety down quickly. However, this means that the anxiety will keep going up to the same level, or maybe higher each time they do a compulsion. Turn to this section of the workbook and share this idea with them with the diagram. Highlight that OCD keeps them in a position where anxiety just keeps going up and down, which must be very uncomfortable. Another thing with OCD, as mentioned earlier, is that the more you do what it wants, the more it keeps adding compulsions to bring anxiety down. Ask them if this has been their experience – whether OCD started off just asking them to do a few compulsions, and then the more they have listened to it, the more compulsions OCD got them to do.

HOW TO BREAK THE OCD CYCLE

Ask the young person if they have ideas on how to break the OCD cycle or things they have tried before. If they say to break the cycle by not facing the triggers of OCD, you can explain that it would be impossible to remove all triggers. If they did manage to avoid triggers, this eventually would lead them to not being able to do lots of things, and we know that OCD will then make them avoid more and more things. They may say they could try to stop the thoughts. If you have not already done so, you can share the 'Learning about thoughts' module in the Appendix in the workbook and in this manual. This highlights that we all get horrible unwanted thoughts and it is difficult to stop them. A helpful exercise to illustrate this point is the pink elephant experiment described in this module. Finally, if they say to stop anxiety, you can ask them if they have ever been told to stop feeling anxious, and what happened? It is likely that they did not experience control over it. You can remind them of what was covered in Session 3, where they learned that we all get anxious and we need that feeling from time to time.

Turn to this section of the workbook, where the OCD cycle of the example of someone checking the door is shared again but this time with the compulsion crossed out. If they have not already shared this as a way to break the OCD cycle, explain that the way to do this is to resist doing what OCD wants – that is, the compulsion. Ask why they think this is the way to break the cycle.

ANXIETY HABITUATION WHEN BREAKING THE OCD CYCLE

Ask them to turn to this section of their workbook to remind them of what happens to anxiety when they face their fears. Explain that they learned with the non-OCD example they shared earlier, that each time they faced their fear, their anxiety reduced and it got easier. This is the same process that happens when facing OCD obsessions and not doing compulsions. Remind them that it does not matter what anxiety-provoking situation they face, anxiety habituation still occurs. Talk them through the anxiety habituation curve using the example of the OCD cycle with checking doors. The first time the person resists checking compulsions they will feel anxious, but their anxiety will go down without them having to do what OCD says. The second time, again anxiety will go up but not as high; the third time, it will be lower and so it goes on.

At this stage, it is helpful to share with the young person that by not doing compulsions, they will learn that anxiety will go down, *and* they will learn to tolerate the uncomfortable feelings. Explain an added bonus of not doing a compulsion is that they may learn something new about their obsession. For example, if the young person stops checking the door repeatedly, they will find out whether someone actually breaks in. Chances are that the likelihood of the feared event is significantly lower than the OCD has been threatening. This can make the obsession become less powerful and eventually it will not pop into their head as much.

THERAPIST NOTE

It is helpful to share that lots of young people with ASD struggle to tolerate strong feelings such as anxiety. They can often find emotions overwhelming, uncontrollable and unpredictable. Let the young person know that by reducing compulsions and facing their fears head on, they can become better able to cope with anxiety and the uncomfortable physical sensations it creates. They can experience for themselves that anxiety is not harmful and does not last forever.

HOMEWORK SESSION 4

Talk through the homework tasks as set out in this section of the workbook. The young person should complete at least two OCD cycles over the week related to their OCD symptoms. They can use their diaries to help them or complete a cycle as it happens during the week. Ask the young person and parent to spend another week completing diaries of OCD symptoms. Explain to them that these will be used in upcoming sessions, so they are very important. Add any unfinished sections from the session for homework.

Session 5

SETTING UP A PLAN

SESSION 5 PLAN

- Set agenda
- Recap of Session 4
- Homework review
- What is ERP?
- OCD hierarchy
- Goals
- Set homework

SET AGENDA

Refer to the workbook and explain to the young person and parent what will be included in the session today. To summarize, share that they will be learning about the main way to challenge OCD using the information they have learned so far, and will think about their goals for treatment.

RECAP: SESSION 4

Spend some time reviewing what was covered in Session 4 to ensure they have understood the contents before moving on today. It is vital they understand the principle of anxiety habituation and how this links to breaking the OCD cycle before moving on in treatment, so do take some time from today's session to revisit this in detail if needed.

HOMEWORK REVIEW

Following on from reviewing the last session, you can examine what they noted as their learning points and address any questions they may have. Check over the OCD cycles they have completed to ensure they have understood how OCD works and see if they have added anything to the OCD diaries this week. Again, if they did not complete homework in this or any future sessions, discuss possible reasons and solutions for this.

WHAT IS ERP?

Explain that today they will be learning about the most important part of treatment for OCD, which is called exposure and response prevention (ERP). This picks up on what was discussed in the last session; it involves facing the triggers of OCD (exposure) and then not doing what OCD wants the young person or other people to do (response prevention). When discussing this, you have an opportunity to reinforce learning from the last session by asking what they think will happen to anxiety when they do ERP.

It is important to highlight at this stage, so this is predictable for the young person with ASD, that they will have to complete an ERP task with you in upcoming sessions and they will practise ERP tasks for homework every week.

Share with the young person that they would never be expected to just resist OCD without a plan, as it can be difficult. Plus, if it was as easy as just resisting OCD, they would have done it by themselves! The plan used to do ERP is called a hierarchy, which is what will be covered next.

OCD HIERARCHY

Share with the young person that in order to know where to start when challenging OCD, developing and using a hierarchy to guide this is helpful. A hierarchy is a list of all the things OCD makes the young person do (compulsions), and avoid or make others do (accommodation). Make sure they add covert or mental compulsions to the list. Anxiety ratings indicating how they would feel if these things were not done or were not avoided because of OCD are used to put the list in order of what is easiest to tackle down to what would be more challenging. This is like a map to know where to go with the ERP tasks.

Invite the young person to use their OCD diaries they completed for homework to list all the things OCD makes them do. Once they have done three to five examples, ask them to list things OCD makes them avoid and things others have to do for OCD. Again, only a few examples of each are needed at this stage. Once they have done this, go through each item in turn and ask the young person how anxious they would feel if they did not do the compulsion, did not avoid the thing or if the other person did not accommodate the OCD. Ask them to look at their anxiety rating scale from Session 3 to aid this process. When using the scale, check whether it is as bad as the non-OCD example they have provided to help anchor their ratings. It can be useful for young people to compare ratings assigned to each compulsion to evaluate which one would be harder or easier – this will help them build their hierarchy. Additionally, it is helpful to remind them of the physical sensations they spoke about related to their anxiety to help with ratings; for example, 'So your breathing would become really fast if you did not do that compulsion?'

The aim in this session is not to complete the entire hierarchy but to ensure that the young person is clear about how to develop a hierarchy – how to list compulsions and generate anxiety ratings. You will ask the young person to complete this for homework, so you need to ensure that they understand the principles.

> **THERAPIST NOTE**
>
> Ensure that behaviours that are added to the hierarchy are compulsions and not ASD repetitive behaviours. Repetitive behaviours may not be unwanted. However, it may be that there are ASD repetitive behaviours or interests that are interfering in life (despite being enjoyable). In such cases, the principles of ERP can be helpful in increasing flexibility and tolerating setting limits around certain behaviours.

GOALS

It is important to spend time with the young person and parent to think about goals for treatment so you all know what they are working towards. It is important to make these SMART – Specific, Measurable, Achievable, Realistic and Time-defined.

Turn to this section of the workbook and ask them to think about goals at set timeframes, for example by the middle of treatment (around Session 10), the end of treatment and in a year's time. For young people with ASD, it is important that these goals are as concrete and specific as possible, so you will see there is a space to add what OCD symptoms would need to be tackled in order to reach the set goal.

It is helpful to get parents involved in the process of supporting the young person to set goals as they will have an insight into how OCD impacts daily life. It is also helpful to see if what the young person and parents want to work towards is the same. If there is a mismatch, this is a useful opportunity to share with the young person that we know OCD impacts them the most, but it can affect everyone (you can share examples from the list of 'What other people do for OCD' to make this point). You may consider, if there is high family accommodation, parents having a list of goals for themselves of things they want to stop doing for OCD.

HOMEWORK SESSION 5

Talk through the homework tasks as set out in this section of the workbook. The young person should complete their OCD hierarchies, including what others have to do for OCD. You may hand over the list of 'What other people do for OCD' to the parent; they can make the list and then the young person can rate how anxious they would feel if their family did not do this for OCD. Explain to the young person that once they have completed their lists and anxiety ratings, they have to put them in order from what makes them least anxious (at the bottom) to most anxious (at the top). This is to put their plan in order, to decide where to start with the OCD challenges (ERP tasks). If the young person did not finish their goals, they can do this for homework, along with anything else they did not complete in session.

Session 6

CHALLENGING OCD USING ERP

SESSION 6 PLAN

- Set agenda
- Recap of Session 5
- Homework review
- CBT for OCD quiz!
- First ERP task!
- Set homework

SET AGENDA

Refer to the workbook and explain to the young person and parent what will be included in the session today. Explain that the focus of the session will be to complete their first ERP task!

RECAP: SESSION 5

Spend some time with the young person and parent to review what was covered in Session 5 to ensure that they have understood the contents before moving on today.

HOMEWORK REVIEW

Following on from reviewing the last session, you can review what they noted as their learning points and address any questions they may have. Review their hierarchies and goals; ensure that the items on their hierarchy cover a range of anxiety ratings as you will need to pick something today for the ERP task. If you notice that all the ratings are very high, you will need to consider breaking the task down.

CBT FOR OCD QUIZ!

To consolidate learning in the sessions so far, complete the true or false quiz in this section of the workbook with the young person and parent. Be vigilant to anything they may not have fully understood at this stage and revisit the relevant sections of the workbook to support their learning.

FIRST ERP TASK!

Explain that in today's session they are going to start challenging OCD and test out all the theory they have learned and put it into practice. Introduce the young person and parent to the worksheet, explaining that this gives a step-by-step plan for how to set up an ERP task. It explains in the workbook that the young person needs their hierarchy to plan a task and anxiety rating scale.

THERAPIST NOTE

Try to bring in the young person's special interests as much as possible to make this process engaging. For example, you can come up with a team name for fighting OCD together, for example 'Doctor Who Fighting the OCD Daleks' or 'Yoda with OCD Missions Each Week'. You can draw out a mission or battle map with various tasks. You can also create reward systems after completing tasks that incorporate their special interests, for example extra time playing Minecraft for every task they complete.

Try to get ERP tasks started early in the session to give the young person a chance to habituate within session. Aim to start the task 15–20 minutes into the session. Before starting the task, ask them to rate how anxious they feel at the moment (Step 1). Young people with ASD often have higher baseline anxiety, so it is important to know this before starting the task. It is helpful information too, as some young people expect their anxiety to come down to the lowest point in the scale. By taking a baseline measure, you can explain to them that you would not expect their anxiety to have gone lower than the level at which it started. You may notice that as you start to discuss the prospect of completing a task, their anxiety may rise above their baseline level (anticipatory anxiety). Explain this is a normal process where anxiety rises in the build-up to doing something scary. This is another reason to try to get the task started as soon as possible. Given anticipatory anxiety, it may be helpful to get a baseline anxiety rating before discussing the task in detail or at the beginning of the session. Ask them to note down their anxiety using their anxiety rating scale from Session 3 of the workbook.

Ask the young person to look at the hierarchy they completed for homework (Session 5) and pick something to challenge today. The aim of this first task is to give them the experience of setting up and undertaking an ERP task successfully. Support the young person to find something on the list that is challenging but manageable. Ideally, it should be something that is practical to complete in the session, but also something they can replicate for homework. It is important to pick something that is a few anxiety points above their baseline anxiety, so they get the experience of their anxiety rising and then habituating back to the baseline within the session.

Once they have picked something, ask them to write it on Step 2 of their ERP task sheet and then consider what obsession this relates to. This could be a specific OCD worry or may be a doubt, just-right feeling or urge. Once this has been identified, ask them to add this to Step 3. In order to reinforce the principles of ERP, Steps 4 and 5 clearly set this out asking the young person to write what the exposure will be (what the trigger is that they will face) and what the response prevention is (what the specific ritual is that they will resist). For young people with ASD, it is important to be very clear and specific, so you should encourage them to add as much information as they can, for example close the front door, walk down the street and not go back. Finally, before starting the ERP task, ask them to predict what they think their anxiety will be. This is helpful to see how accurate their predictions are and notice patterns in this, for example do they always predict that anxiety will be higher than it is.

Explain that they will track their anxiety during the task to see what happens. Encourage the young person to start their task. As soon as they have completed the exposure and resisted the ritual completely, use the anxiety rating scale to help them to rate their anxiety at the 0 minute time point. For young people with ASD, you may need to support this process further by asking them to focus on one or more of the physical sensations in their body and notice changes in the specific feeling.

Track the anxiety at the various time points on the worksheet. You may run out of time in the session, so encourage the young person and parent to continue to track this after the session has ended. It may be helpful, in addition to the young person writing down their ratings, to draw this out on a board in the form of a graph so it can be compared to the habituation graph in their workbook (Session 4).

Typically, the task is complete when the anxiety has gone back to the baseline anxiety point or if the amount of anxiety they have experienced has halved, whichever of the two is higher; for example, if their baseline was three and the task took it up to an eight, the task would be over when it is down to a four, which is higher than the baseline of three. Congratulate the young person in completing their first task - even if they ended up doing a ritual or the anxiety has not yet habituated, they should be congratulated for trying.

Be careful in sessions that conversation during or after tasks does not become a form of distraction. It is important that the young person focuses on their anxiety symptoms in order to learn that they can tolerate the feeling and to fully experience the process of habituation. If you notice that conversation brings anxiety down quickly or they are not focusing on the anxiety in the session, you may need to develop rules for tasks, such as no talking after tasks or sitting in silence.

THERAPIST NOTE

There are several things to consider when undertaking ERP tasks with young people with ASD:

- It is important to not start too high on the hierarchy as people with ASD may struggle with distress tolerance.
- They may struggle to predict their anxiety for tasks – finding it easier or more difficult than predicted. It is useful to use parents to help gauge what may be appropriate tasks.
- If they are struggling to come up with a task, you may find it helpful to link it directly to their goals as a way to make it concrete and meaningful.
- If they refuse to do a task, explore why this may be the case; it may be due to anxiety, so think about steps they can do to break the task down and build up to it to increase their confidence. If they express that they do not see the point of the task, link the task to their goals.
- If the young person is struggling to complete ERP tasks, you may wish to consider you or the parent modelling the task first, so the young person knows what to do. This may be particularly helpful for young people with ASD as it gives them a concrete representation of what they are required to do. Be careful this does not become a form of reassurance, for example they want to see if anything bad happens to the person modelling the task before they do it. To test this out, try in future tasks to mix up whether they are modelled or not to see if this affects the young person's anxiety level and explore with them whether tasks felt easier if modelled and if this is providing OCD with reassurance.
- If their anxiety is higher than they predicted, you may have to accommodate the OCD the first time and then think about how to break the task down further into manageable steps.
- It often takes longer for anxiety to habituate in those with ASD, therefore it may still be high at the end of the session. If this happens, advise their parent to support them to track their anxiety levels after the session has ended. This is important as it highlights the expectation that habituation will occur and promotes learning that ERP tasks continue outside the sessions. In doing this, it is important to consider whether distraction after the session will lead to their

anxiety reducing. If this is the case, encourage the family to think of ways to manage this, such as sitting in the waiting area quietly while monitoring anxiety.

- For some young people with ASD, the anxiety is largely anticipatory and so you may see the anxiety quickly come down after ERP. If you are confident that this is not as a result of completing any compulsions, then just encourage the young person to think about what they have learned and how they can continue to practise this.
- Sometimes anxiety does not get triggered by the task; consider if they did feel anxious but did not recognize it (if you see physical signs of anxiety it may be helpful to share these with the young person), they did a compulsion (maybe a covert ritual) to bring the anxiety down or they were distracted during the task. If any of these are the case, they would need to be tackled in the next task. If none of these reasons are relevant, it may be that the next task needs to be higher on their hierarchy.
- As mentioned above, be careful of distraction in sessions. Young people with ASD may need rules on what to do during and after tasks, such as to sit in silence and focus on anxiety symptoms. They will need rules on what to do when they leave the session, such as not to do compulsions later. If compulsions are daily activities like washing hands, as long as this happens after anxiety has habituated and not in response to OCD obsessions, this is okay.
- Some young people with ASD may rate how strong their thoughts or worries are instead of the physiological signs of anxiety. Support the young person to zoom into one or two physical indicators of anxiety and prompt them to keep focusing on this to support them with ratings.
- Be mindful of ASD sensory sensitivities during ERP tasks; some young people may not like the smell, sound or touch of things, for example the smell of metal when touching door handles, which they also see as contaminated because of OCD. It is helpful to consider and highlight when setting up ERP tasks that two areas are likely to be tackled in such tasks: OCD and tolerating the anxiety/discomfort associated with sensory sensitivities. You may wish to consider rating OCD-related anxiety and sensory sensitivity discomfort separately in such tasks, as each may habituate at different rates. If this feels too complicated for the young person, it is important to highlight that their anxiety rating is made up of the two elements to acknowledge why ratings may be higher or it may take longer to habituate.
- Some people with ASD may exhibit high levels of anxiety in the form of aggressive behaviour, self-harm, running away and so on. As well as this being an indication of the task needing to be broken down into manageable steps, you may need to consider supporting the family in managing certain behaviours

(e.g. kicking, swearing, etc.) should these be considered not acceptable even while the person is experiencing heightened anxiety during ERP tasks. Think together about how this would be typically managed in the family and if this is an appropriate response, and encourage the parent to respond in the same way to this in the context of tasks. Share this with the young person so this is clear and predictable for them.

- Young people with ASD may need additional strategies to support them to get their baseline anxiety lower. See the 'Managing ASD-related stress' optional module for more details (in the Appendix of this manual).
- We know other people get pulled into doing things for OCD and will be asked to challenge this in treatment (see 'Ask others to challenge OCD' in Appendix). For young people with ASD, it is crucial that there is consistency across individuals and settings in how OCD is responded to. Therefore, it will be important to involve other systems (e.g. school) in their treatment and provide guidance on how they respond to OCD, and when and how to challenge OCD depending on what tasks are being completed in sessions. In the same way parents are given feedback on sessions and informed on homework tasks, it may be helpful for others to know the same information so they can support the young person to engage in ERP tasks across settings.

HOMEWORK SESSION 6

Talk through the homework tasks as set out in this section of the workbook. The young person should continue to add to their OCD hierarchies with any new compulsions, things they avoid or what others have to do for OCD over the week. In setting up the ERP task today, you have hopefully chosen something that can be repeated in exactly the same way for homework. Ask the young person to practise the task at least once a day and note their anxiety. There is a timetable in the workbook for them to use to help schedule their ERP homework tasks.

Session 7

CHALLENGING OCD USING ERP (AND OCD REVIEW)

SESSION 7 PLAN

- Set agenda
- Recap of Session 6
- Homework review
- Review OCD
- ERP task!
- Set homework

SET AGENDA

Refer to the workbook and explain to the young person and parent what will be covered. To summarize what is happening in the session, explain that you will be reviewing OCD and undertaking another ERP task.

RECAP: SESSION 6

Spend some time with the young person and parent to review what was covered in Session 6 to ensure that they have understood the contents before moving on today.

HOMEWORK REVIEW

As always, you will review what the young person noted as their learning points from the last session and address any questions they may have. It is important to spend some time looking over the ERP task recordings for the week. If they managed to complete the task every day, invite them to reflect on what happened to their anxiety over time and each time they practised the task. If they completed it as planned, they may have noticed their anxiety habituated and it got easier each time, and they learned to tolerate the uncomfortable feelings. If this is the case, ask them to complete Step 9 on the ERP task sheet to state what they have learned about anxiety by doing this task and if they learned anything about their obsession (this may be unlikely at this stage).

If they did not complete ERP tasks at least once a day, ask why this was the case and try to consider ways forward together. Explain that moving forward with ERP tasks will be the main part of homework, so finding a way to do these at home every day is important. Invite the parent to share their ideas and thoughts.

THERAPIST NOTE

You may find the young person reports that their anxiety remained high over the course of the week. Ask if they have noticed other rituals creeping in, if they were distracting themselves, giving themselves reassurance or their family were doing things to bring their anxiety down. During the tasks for homework and in the session, it is important to look out for subtle rituals that may be undermining the ERP task. If you notice that their anxiety is coming down quickly or suddenly, enquire if there may be mental rituals they are completing or whether OCD is making them do anything else to make the anxiety come down. It is important to keep an eye on what the family might be doing during the task – do they try to do something to reduce the anxiety like give them reassurance by saying, 'Don't worry, nothing bad will happen'? If this is the case, refer to the module 'Ask others to challenge OCD' (see the Appendix in the workbook and in this manual).

Bring this back to the OCD cycle (Session 4 of the workbook) to highlight that anxiety usually stays high due to compulsions, so they have to look out for this when undertaking tasks. Explore this with the young person and parent, and if it is agreed that something is bringing the anxiety down quickly, like a ritual, it should be added to the hierarchy to be challenged. The aim is to support the young person to learn they can tolerate anxiety without needing to do anything to reduce it. Congratulate them for making the effort to complete tasks and externalize the difficulties in conducting tasks due to OCD playing tricks!

REVIEW OCD

Remind the young person and parent that there are regular reviews during CBT to ensure that the treatment is working. Assure them at this stage we would not expect a big change in their OCD as we know ERP tasks are the main way to challenge OCD and they have only been doing this for a week. It is important to get an up-to-date measure, so everyone knows how things are at present.

Administer the measure you completed at assessment and plot this on the graph in the workbook. If there has been an increase in symptoms, this can be normalized as we know OCD can get worse so long as compulsions are completed. You can explore other reasons for why this may be the case, such as high levels of anxiety generally, the stress of starting treatment and so on. It is also possible that talking more about the symptoms may have led to them becoming more aware of the impact of OCD. If the score has reduced, explore with the young person how they think this has happened. Listen out for anything they say that fits with the ERP model and breaking the OCD cycle and share this with them.

ERP TASK!

As in Session 6, the young person will complete an ERP task following the same steps they completed last time. If they were successful in completing the task in session and for homework, you can consider building on this task. Alternatively, you can review their hierarchy and pick the next thing on their OCD hierarchy to challenge. Before the session ends, ensure that they have completed anxiety ratings and that any learning from the ERP task today is added to Step 9 in the workbook.

HOMEWORK SESSION 7

Talk through the homework tasks as set out in the workbook. The young person should continue to add to their OCD hierarchies with any new compulsions, things they avoid or what others have to do for OCD that they notice over the week. Ask them to keep practising their ERP task from Session 6 and today's ERP task every day. Explain that the more they practise, the easier it will get. Use the timetable in the workbook to help them to schedule their ERP homework tasks.

Session 8

CHALLENGING OCD USING ERP

SESSION 8 PLAN

- Set agenda
- Recap of Session 7
- Homework review
- ERP task!
- OCD steps
- Set homework

SET AGENDA

Refer to the workbook and explain to the young person and parent what will be included in the session today. Explain that they will complete another ERP challenge and you will introduce something they can use to help them with the task.

RECAP: SESSION 7

Spend some time with the young person and parent to review what was covered in Session 7 to ensure they have understood the contents before moving on today.

HOMEWORK REVIEW

Review what the young person noted as their learning points from the last session and address any questions they may have. Review ERP tasks in the same way as in the previous session, adding any learning from tasks on Step 9 of the ERP task sheet. If the young person has struggled to do tasks, you can share that one reason may be because they felt too challenging. Explain that in today's session, they will be given a worksheet to help them with this.

ERP TASK!

Today, the young person will complete an ERP task following the same steps they completed last week. You can review their hierarchy and pick the next thing or continue to build on the tasks they have already completed. An alternative, and something that is helpful to use for young people with ASD, are the OCD steps in the workbook (see below for an explanation of how to use these).

THERAPIST NOTE

Now you have an idea of what is included on the hierarchy, think with the young person and family about tasks in future sessions and whether they need to bring things into the session to trigger OCD. You may need to consider leaving the clinic setting, including incorporating home visits. It is important for young people with ASD that the tasks are as realistic as possible, and it is helpful to do the tasks in settings where OCD typically gets triggered, to help them generalize learning from tasks in sessions to real-life situations.

OCD STEPS

When a young person is finding the tasks on their hierarchy challenging, they can use the OCD steps to break down the task into smaller, more manageable targets – each item on the hierarchy can be broken down into mini-steps. An alternative or additional way these steps can be used is to come up with a plan to reach a specific goal. At the top, the young person can write the ritual they want to resist or the goal they want to work towards. In the bottom step, ask the young person to write what they are doing at the moment. Support the young person to think through what steps they would need to take to get from where they are now to where they would like to be (at the top). Ask them to rate how anxious they would feel at each step. You may come back to review the anxiety ratings in future sessions as they move through the steps, as they may notice their anxiety predictions will change as they progress through the steps. These steps are included throughout the workbook and can be used any time you think it would be helpful to include in a session.

THERAPIST NOTE

Young people with ASD often find it difficult to understand how individual ERP tasks relate to their everyday life. It can be difficult for them to generalize their learning from the challenges in the sessions to their goals at home. Where possible, support the young person to specifically link the ERP to one of their main goals. This may help to make their tasks feel more meaningful and targeted. It may also help boost their motivation.

THERAPIST NOTE

While the goal is to resist compulsions altogether to break the OCD cycle, young people with ASD may struggle to do this at first, so you could consider some interim strategies to support them. For example:

- Delaying rituals, e.g. delaying handwashing by increasing increments each time they face a trigger.
- Completing a ritual but not exactly how OCD wants them to, for example washing hands four times instead of doing it five times.
- Using techniques such as distraction to make the anxiety more tolerable in the short term, for example playing a game after the task.

It is important to share with the young person that these are only short-term measures. Eventually, we will support them to resist the compulsion altogether; this is just a way to help them get there. You can use the OCD steps to write out what the plan is, with the goal being to resist the ritual completely.

HOMEWORK SESSION 8

Talk through the homework tasks as set out in this section of the workbook. The young person should continue to add to their OCD hierarchies with any new compulsions, things they avoid or what others have to do for OCD that they notice over the week. Ask them to keep practising every day their ERP tasks from Sessions 6, 7 and today. Explain that the more they practise, the easier it will get. Use the downloadable timetable in the workbook to help them to schedule their ERP homework tasks.

Session 9

CHALLENGING OCD USING ERP

SESSION 9 PLAN

- Set agenda
- Recap of Session 8
- Homework review
- ERP task!
- Things to help you to do ERP
- Set homework

SET AGENDA

Refer to the workbook and explain to the young person and parent what will be included in the session today. They will complete an ERP task and you will discuss additional things they can do to help them complete the tasks.

RECAP: SESSION 8

Spend some time with the young person and parent to review what was covered in Session 8 to ensure that they have understood the contents before moving on today.

HOMEWORK REVIEW

Review what they noted as their learning points from the last session and address any questions they may have. Review ERP tasks in the same way as in previous sessions, adding learning from tasks to Step 9 of the ERP task sheet.

ERP TASK!

As in previous sessions, today the young person will complete an ERP task following the same steps. You can review their hierarchy/OCD steps and pick the next thing or continue to build on the tasks they have already completed.

THINGS TO HELP YOU DO ERP

You will see in the workbook that there are suggestions of things that may help support the young person to undertake ERP tasks. Some ideas are on the page while others are detailed in the Appendix. One idea shared on this page is that the young person can take photos or videos of their tasks. This can be a valuable visual reminder of tasks young people with ASD have completed. If and when they are struggling with tasks during treatment, you can refer to pictures or videos to remind them of all the hard work they have already done.

Another suggestion is to keep a diary of every time they have beaten OCD. They are already keeping records of their anxiety ratings, but you can be creative and find other ways to record their achievements, with the focus on what they have beaten. This could involve having post-it notes of everything they have accomplished put in places that trigger OCD, or a record on their phone, as well as a physical diary.

Rewards can be a powerful way to encourage the young person to engage with ERP tasks. Given that the experience of ERP can be aversive and many young people with ASD may lack insight into their OCD or not understand the reason to engage in ERP tasks, incorporating a reward system into tasks may be beneficial. These do not need to be tangible goods but could include extra time for their special interests or enjoyable activities with their family. They should get rewards for attempting the tasks and facing their fears, as opposed to the outcome of the task, for example whether they habituate or not. When using a reward system, it is helpful to check the young person's understanding of why they are doing tasks and how it links to getting better from OCD, to avoid them just focusing on the reward. If they struggle to understand this, support the parent to share this with them.

Other suggestions are included in the Appendix of the workbook and of this manual.

THERAPIST NOTE

Young people with ASD often experience higher levels of baseline anxiety, which can sometimes make their ability to undertake ERP tasks or move up the hierarchy more challenging. It can be helpful to augment the treatment with additional tools to help manage ASD-related stress to reduce their baseline anxiety (see 'Managing ASD-related stress' in the Appendix of this manual).

HOMEWORK SESSION 9

Talk through the homework tasks as set out in this section of the workbook. The young person and family should look out for new compulsions, things they avoid or what others have to do for OCD that they notice over the week. Ask them to keep practising today's ERP task daily, alongside their tasks from previous sessions. Explain that the more they practise, the easier it will get. Use the downloadable timetable in the workbook to help them to schedule their ERP homework tasks.

THERAPIST NOTE

When a task is starting to be easy and does not make the young person feel anxious anymore, you can consider taking it off the daily practice list. This refers to tasks that are in addition to daily activities, such as an ERP task of purposely touching the bin, rather than tasks that should become part of daily life, like washing hands for a shorter period. Taking these tasks off their list will prevent the young person feeling overwhelmed with homework tasks. However, be cautious and check in on any compulsions that have come off the list from time to time, to ensure they do not sneak back in again and become a problem. It may help to ask them to practise the task on and off over the course of the treatment. It is helpful to share this as a rule for young people with ASD. To support generalization and to ensure that there is ongoing challenging of OCD, you can ask the young person and family what they should now be able to do given they have challenged a compulsion that is coming off their practice list – for example, the touching bin task now means they can put rubbish in the bin and not wash hands afterwards.

Session 10

CHALLENGING OCD USING ERP

SESSION 10 PLAN

- Set agenda
- Recap of Session 9
- Homework review
- ERP task!
- Set homework

SET AGENDA

Refer to the workbook and explain to the young person and parent what will be included in the session today. Explain that the focus will be on the ERP task.

RECAP: SESSION 9

Spend some time with the young person and parent to review what was covered in Session 9 to ensure that they have understood the contents before moving on today.

HOMEWORK REVIEW

Review what they noted as their learning points from the last session and address any questions they may have. Check if they have added anything new to their hierarchies. Review ERP tasks in the same way as in previous sessions, adding anything they learned following their tasks to Step 9 on the ERP task sheet.

ERP TASK!

As in previous sessions, today the young person will complete an ERP task following the same steps. You can review their hierarchy/OCD steps and pick the next thing or continue to build on the tasks they have already completed.

THERAPIST NOTE

Note that there is an extra step added to the ERP task sheet in this part of the workbook; Step 7 is now asking the young person whether they need anything to help them do the ERP task. This may include what was discussed last week (e.g. photos, rewards charts) and you may wish to revisit some ideas. After Step 10 (reflecting on learning), there are additional questions asking, now that they have completed the task, what other tasks might be similar to this? This serves to support the young person to start generalizing between tasks, which we know young people with ASD struggle to do; for example, now they can resist checking plugs at the clinic, they can do it at home. The young person is also encouraged to think about how the task they have completed in the session links to things they can now do in day-to-day life; for example, if they are not repeatedly checking the door, they can get to school on time.

HOMEWORK SESSION 10

Talk through the homework tasks as set out in this section of the workbook. Ask them to keep practising today's ERP task daily, alongside their tasks from previous sessions. Explain that the more they practise, the easier it will get. Use the downloadable timetable in the workbook to help schedule their ERP homework tasks.

Session 11

CHALLENGING OCD USING ERP

SESSION 11 PLAN

- Set agenda
- Recap of Session 10
- Homework review
- ERP task!
- Set homework

SET AGENDA

Refer to the workbook and explain to the young person and parent what will be included in the session today. Explain that the focus will be on the ERP task.

RECAP: SESSION 10

Spend some time with the young person and parent to review what was covered in Session 10 to ensure that they have understood the contents before moving on today.

HOMEWORK REVIEW

As always, you will review what they noted as their learning points from the last session and address any questions they may have. Review ERP tasks in the same way as in previous sessions, adding anything they learned by completing tasks to Step 10 on the ERP task sheet.

THERAPIST NOTE

If you have noticed that the young person is not completing ERP tasks consistently, and none of the suggestions for how to overcome this have worked, you may need to share with the young person and parent that it is unlikely treatment will be effective. Think together about ways this can be addressed and consider if a break in therapy is needed and to come back to this when they are ready. You could ask them to consider whether the family reducing their accommodations is worth considering as a way forward if the young person is struggling to do tasks themselves. Ongoing sessions can be used to focus on family accommodation using the workbook in the same way. It can be helpful to keep the young person involved in these sessions, so they are aware of the plans being made, to ensure predictability. You can focus on the 'What other people do for OCD' hierarchy (Session 5 of the workbook). These parts of the treatment workbook can also be used if you are noticing that family members are struggling to disengage from doing what OCD wants.

ERP TASK!

As in previous sessions, today the young person will complete an ERP task following the same steps. You can review their hierarchy/OCD steps and pick the next thing or continue to build on the tasks they have already completed.

HOMEWORK SESSION 11

Talk through the homework tasks as set out in this section of the workbook. The young person should keep practising their ERP tasks from today and previous sessions every day. Explain that the more they practise, the easier it will get. Use the downloadable timetable in the workbook to help them schedule their ERP homework tasks.

Session 12

CHALLENGING OCD USING ERP

SESSION 12 PLAN

- Set agenda
- Recap of Session 11
- Homework review
- ERP task!
- Rules for challenging OCD
- Set homework

SET AGENDA

Refer to the workbook and explain to the young person and parent what will be included in the session today. They will be completing another ERP task and thinking about some rules to challenge OCD.

RECAP: SESSION 11

Spend some time with the young person and parent to review what was covered in Session 11 to ensure that they have understood the contents before moving on today.

HOMEWORK REVIEW

As always, you will review what they noted as their learning points from the last session and address any questions they may have. Review ERP tasks in the same way as in previous sessions, adding anything they learned by completing tasks to Step 10 on the ERP task sheet.

ERP TASK!

As in previous sessions, today the young person will complete an ERP task following the same steps. You can review their hierarchy/OCD steps and pick the next thing or continue to build on the tasks they have already completed.

THERAPIST NOTE

If the young person is doing well with their ERP tasks (i.e. moving up their hierarchy, tolerating anxiety, experiencing habituation), you can consider whether they may be able to take some bigger jumps up their hierarchy. Young people with ASD may struggle with what seems like a change in rule. You can explain that this may help speed up their recovery if they skip some steps and move higher up. They can do the lower steps for homework and they are more likely to be able to achieve the lower steps as they have completed harder tasks in sessions. This will allow you to focus sessions on doing the challenging tasks. It may be helpful to draw out similarities between tasks they have completed in the sessions with homework tasks; for example, if they managed to do something that is a seven on their anxiety rating scale, could they try other tasks they rated as seven at home? You can draw up some amended rules if this is a way the young person is happy to move forward, highlighting that the ERP principles are exactly the same.

RULES FOR CHALLENGING OCD

To promote further generalization of learning, the young person and parent are invited to share the key rules for challenging OCD. This is completed at this stage of treatment, not only to consolidate their experiences and learning to date, but also to prepare the family for setting up their own ERP tasks in future sessions. These rules apply no matter what OCD makes them or others do or makes them avoid. Examples of helpful learning points might be to:

- use the hierarchy/OCD steps to decide what to challenge
- do ERP tasks as much as possible (at least daily)
- keep doing ERP tasks until they become easy/feel less scary
- move up the hierarchy/OCD steps
- listen to parents giving reminders to do tasks at home
- remember that OCD doesn't tell the truth – it's not usually as bad as they think it's going to be!

HOMEWORK SESSION 12

Talk through the homework tasks as set out in this section of the workbook. The young person should keep practising their ERP tasks from today and previous sessions every day, and they may be adding tasks that have not been completed in session to their list at this stage. Use the downloadable timetable in the workbook to help them to schedule their ERP homework tasks.

You will notice that for homework, instead of thinking about what they learned in the session today, they will now be encouraged to think about what they have learned in treatment so far. This aims to promote generalization and to reinforce their rules for challenging OCD.

Session 13

CHALLENGING OCD USING ERP

SESSION 13 PLAN

- Set agenda
- Recap of Session 12
- Homework review
- ERP task!
- Set homework

SET AGENDA

Refer to the workbook and explain to the young person and parent what will be included in the session today. Explain that the focus of the session will be on doing an ERP task.

RECAP: SESSION 12

Spend some time with the young person and parent to review what was covered in Session 12 to ensure they have understood the contents before moving on today. Explain that the focus will be on ERP.

HOMEWORK REVIEW

As always, you will review what they noted as their learning points from treatment so far and address any questions they may have. Review ERP tasks in the same way as in previous sessions, adding learning from tasks to Step 10 on the ERP task sheet.

ERP TASK!

Like in previous sessions, today the young person will complete an ERP task following the same steps. You can review their hierarchy/OCD steps and pick the next thing or continue to build on the tasks they have already completed.

HOMEWORK SESSION 13

Talk through the homework tasks as set out in this section of the workbook. The young person should keep practising their ERP tasks from today and previous sessions every day, and they may be adding tasks that have not been completed in session to their list at this stage. Use the downloadable timetable in the workbook to help them to schedule their ERP homework tasks.

Session 14

CHALLENGING OCD USING ERP (AND OCD REVIEW)

SESSION 14 PLAN

- Set agenda
- Recap of Session 13
- Homework review
- Review OCD
- ERP task!
- Set homework

SET AGENDA

Refer to the workbook and explain to the young person and parent what will be included in the session today. Explain that the focus will be to take a measure of OCD to review progress and complete an ERP task.

RECAP: SESSION 13

Spend some time with the young person and parent to review what was covered in Session 13 to ensure they have understood the contents before moving on today.

HOMEWORK REVIEW

As always, you will review what they noted as their learning points from treatment so far and address any questions they may have. Review ERP tasks in the same way as in previous sessions, adding any learning from tasks to Step 10 on the ERP task sheet.

REVIEW OCD

Remind the young person and parent that there are regular reviews during CBT to ensure that the treatment is working. Administer the measure you completed at assessment and Session 7, and plot this on the graph in the workbook. If the score has reduced, explore with the young person how they think this has happened. Listen out for anything they say that fits with the ERP model and breaking the OCD cycle and share this with them. Ask them to reflect on progress and set out what they still have to work on in the remaining sessions, referring to the goals they set themselves.

If the score remains the same or has worsened since Session 7, explore the reasons for this with the young person and parent. If they have been inconsistent in completing ERP tasks or are not moving up their hierarchy, this could be suggested as a possible reason for why their OCD is not improving. Share this with them and explore if there are ways to move this forward.

There may be many reasons for lack of progress in sessions as well as not completing consistent and daily ERP tasks. One reason is that a young person may not have been able to disclose an obsession to you in session as yet, so it has not been tackled. This may be because they are ashamed and embarrassed, or worry that they may get into trouble if they tell you, or they think if they say it, it will come true. You can again share this with the young person and try to find ways to help them disclose this to you, for example using the 'Learning about thoughts' module (see the Appendix in the workbook and in this manual) to share surveys of normal intrusive thoughts and to learn about the power of thoughts. You may suggest that the parent leaves the room if this will make it easier for the young person to disclose an issue, or you could ask them to write it down. It is important to stress to them that if you do not know what is going on, you cannot help them overcome this.

As mentioned earlier, subtle or mental rituals may be undermining tasks they are completing, or OCD may be making them engage in compensatory rituals after sessions to make up for the ERP tasks. Parents may have slipped into accommodating OCD in other ways or be giving the young person reassurance, which again would undermine the ERP tasks. It is important to support them to recognize this and for anything identified to be added to the hierarchy, so it can be challenged.

ERP TASK!

As in previous sessions, today the young person will complete an ERP task following the same steps. You can review their hierarchy/OCD steps and pick the next thing or continue to build on the tasks they have already completed. Before the session ends, ensure that the young person has completed their anxiety ratings and that any learning from the ERP task today is added to Step 10 in the workbook. Remind the family that in the next session they will be leading on the ERP task.

HOMEWORK SESSION 14

Talk through the homework tasks as set out in this section of the workbook. The young person should keep practising their ERP tasks from today and previous sessions every day, and they may be adding tasks that have not been completed in session to their list at this stage. Use the downloadable timetable in the workbook to help them to schedule their ERP homework tasks. The young person should also be asked to go through their hierarchy to see what is left to tackle and to do their anxiety ratings again as they may have changed.

SESSIONS 15–18

CHALLENGING OCD USING ERP – YOU TAKE CHARGE

SESSIONS 15–18 PLAN

- Set agenda
- Recap of previous session
- Homework review
- ERP task!
- Things to help you do ERP
- Set homework

SET AGENDA

Refer to the workbook and explain to the young person and parent what will be included in the session today. Explain that the focus on the session will be on ERP (and thinking through any ideas of things that can help them to do ERP) and on them taking charge of setting up and doing the task.

RECAP: PREVIOUS SESSION

Spend some time with the young person and parent to review what was covered in the previous session to ensure that they have understood the contents before moving on today.

HOMEWORK REVIEW

As always, you will review what they noted as their learning points from treatment so far and address any questions they may have. It is important to spend some time looking over the ERP task recordings for the week. Invite them to reflect on what happened to their anxiety over time and each time they practise tasks. If they completed a task as planned, they would have noticed their anxiety would have habituated and it got easier each time. Ask them to add any new learning to Step 10 on the ERP task sheet in their workbook. It is important for them to think about what they are learning about their obsession.

ERP TASK!

As in previous sessions, today the young person will complete an ERP task following the same steps. You can review their hierarchy/OCD steps and pick the next thing or continue to build on the tasks they have already completed. However, you will ask the young person and parent to take the lead in this and set up the task with minimal input from you. Ask them to follow the ERP sheets as they usually would but also to refer to the rules for challenging OCD (Session 12) to help them with this.

Explain the rationale for them taking a lead is to prepare them for when weekly sessions end, so they can build confidence in knowing what they have to do. They should have completed lots of ERP tasks in session and for homework now, so they should be well prepared for this next stage.

Your role is to try to step back and observe the process of the family setting up and undertaking tasks. If you have the facilities, you can observe from another room or ensure that you are sitting back from the family to allow them to focus on the task. It is helpful for you to take notes on what steps in setting up the tasks they did well and what may need improving; for example, could they have pushed harder with the task? Did you notice any compulsions creeping in? Arrange some time in the session to ask the young person what they felt went well and what could be improved on before sharing your feedback. Give lots of encouragement and praise for any steps they are taking that are in line with what you have been doing in treatment so far, and add ideas if they are struggling or if you think they should be doing something differently, such as choosing a more difficult task in the hierarchy.

If the young person and parent are lacking confidence in planning and conducting their own ERP tasks, you can develop a hierarchy with them about how to reduce your involvement and increase their autonomy step by step over the next four sessions. For example, as a first step, you could help them pick the task on the hierarchy but they then complete the task; then the next step is for you to give them two options of tasks and they make the final decision and do the task; this finally moves towards them choosing and completing tasks without your input.

THINGS TO HELP YOU DO ERP

This is included again in Session 15 of the workbook but can be used at any point during the ERP phase of treatment if you feel it would be helpful. Refer to the Appendix in the workbook and in this manual for the modules. You may have additional ideas to add to this.

If it is difficult to devise ERP tasks in-vivo, such as facing fears of going to hell or their parent dying, or to find creative ways to develop ERP tasks, there are various options to try out. One way to tackle this is to use imaginal exposure; here you could ask the young person to imagine being in their feared situation to elicit the same fear the obsession creates – ask them to describe or write down a detailed description of being in hell and do the ERP task with that as the trigger. Another way to expose to the obsession is to use loop tapes. Here the young person records the obsessions in the way OCD says it to them, for example 'You will go to hell', and they listen to this over and over again until their anxiety triggered by the thoughts reduces. You can use dictaphones or their mobile phones to create this. The principle of ERP is the same – for them to listen to the loop tape (exposure) and to resist compulsions (response prevention). As with all ERP tasks, it is important to be vigilant to any covert rituals during imaginal tasks. Loop tapes can also be used during ERP tasks when they can face the trigger in the session to make the tasks more challenging; for example, someone who has resisted checking that the door is locked can listen to a recording saying their house will be broken into. Some therapists and parents become concerned about exposure to thoughts. It is important to remember that the young person is frequently experiencing these thoughts and this gives them a chance to experience them without doing rituals to reduce the distress they cause. These thoughts are what they are experiencing anyway. You can also test out the power of thoughts in sessions (please refer to the module 'Learning about thoughts' in the Appendix of the workbook and of this manual).

HOMEWORK SESSIONS 15–18

The focus of homework in these sessions is practising as many ERP tasks as possible for homework, with a mixture of what they have completed in session and tasks they have not set up in session. This gives them opportunities to practise planning and undertaking tasks independently in preparation for weekly sessions ending. Encourage them to keep linking what they are doing to the rules to challenge OCD they devised and the goals they are working towards.

Session 19

CHALLENGING OCD USING ERP AND GETTING READY FOR THE FINISH

SESSION 19 PLAN

- Set agenda
- Recap of Session 18
- Homework review
- ERP or extreme task!
- Getting ready for the finish
- Set homework

SET AGENDA

Refer to the workbook and explain to the young person and parent what will be included in the session. Explain that today the focus will be on completing the final ERP task in session and to start to plan for weekly sessions coming to an end.

RECAP: SESSION 18

Spend some time with the young person and parent to review what was covered in Session 18 to ensure they have understood the contents before moving on today.

HOMEWORK REVIEW

Review what they noted as their learning points and address any questions they may have. Review ERP tasks as you have been doing through treatment, but with a focus on thinking about their confidence in setting up and conducting ERP tasks independently. If they have had any issues with that, spend some time supporting them to think about ways to overcome obstacles. Congratulate them if they have been doing well with this.

ERP OR EXTREME TASK!

As this is the final session where the young person has the chance to do an ERP task, they can be given the option of completing an 'extreme' task or an 'overlearning' task. The steps in setting the task up are the same as with other ERP tasks, but it involves going beyond what is typical in day-to-day life to really tackle the obsession. This is to show OCD that they have really overcome their fear. The focus of completing the task is less on habituation but rather on showing OCD who is boss. The type of tasks may include eating a piece of food from a toilet seat if they had contamination concerns or leaving their windows open if they were worried about a break-in. Consider if this is a task where some modelling (from you or their parent) would be helpful. If this is something you are considering doing in this session, you may wish to mention this in advance, so they can start thinking of ideas. There is a worksheet called 'Extreme tasks' in the Appendix of the workbook to help you plan out the overlearning task.

If the young person is unsure about completing an extreme overlearning task, you can continue with an ERP task but should try to maximize the opportunity of the last task by trying to go as high on their hierarchy as they can manage. Again, this gives them a good final in-session experience of victory over OCD.

GETTING READY FOR THE FINISH

Once the task is under way, you can start to think with the young person about next steps after completing their weekly CBT sessions. Be mindful of this conversation potentially being a distraction from the task, and if this is the case, have this conversation before the ERP task. There are a series of questions for them to complete, encouraging them to review their successes and to see what OCD symptoms they have been able to challenge in CBT. There is an opportunity for them to share how they managed to overcome these symptoms and the rules they have used for challenging OCD. It may be that they still have OCD symptoms left to work on, so they are asked to write these down and set up a plan for how to do this.

Remember to keep monitoring their anxiety for today's ERP task and to write down their learning before the session is completed.

HOMEWORK SESSION 19

The young person should continue with engaging and practising ERP tasks that they have completed to date but should be adding new tasks to the list. They are encouraged to read over the content of the next session in preparation for developing a relapse prevention plan. They have timetables they can download to plan their tasks. They are also asked to reflect on their learning in treatment.

Session 20

RELAPSE PREVENTION PLAN

SESSION 20 PLAN

- Set agenda
- Recap of Session 19
- Homework review
- Relapse prevention plan
- Review OCD
- Planning ahead
- Certificate

SET AGENDA

Refer to the workbook and explain to the young person and parent what will be included in the session today. Explain that they will develop a relapse prevention plan and plan ahead to their review appointment. They will complete a measure of their OCD to review progress.

RECAP: SESSION 19

Spend some time with the young person and parent to review what was covered in Session 19 to ensure that they have understood the contents before moving on today.

HOMEWORK REVIEW

Review the ERP tasks they completed since the last session, reflecting on their learning from the tasks and how they will take them forward. Ask them to add any new learning to Step 10 on the ERP task sheet in their workbook. Enquire if they have read over Session 20 in their workbook in preparation for today's session and if they have any questions.

RELAPSE PREVENTION PLAN

Turn to this section of their workbook. Congratulate the young person and their parent on all the hard work and effort they have put into treatment. Look back at the goals they set themselves at the end of treatment (Session 5 in the workbook) and explore their progress towards these targets. It is important to explain that even though weekly sessions are ending, the work still continues. This is why they have been taking a lead with their tasks in sessions, to prepare them to continue their OCD fighting independently. They may have achieved what they wanted to, which is great, and now the focus is about using what they know about how to challenge OCD to keep it away.

Ask them to think about what they have overcome, and to think about what might be triggers for those symptoms to come back. Ask them to consider any changes or any events they may find stressful that are coming up in the foreseeable future and to add this to the box. We know that OCD tends to worsen when young people feel stressed, tired or ill. If they know this, they can be prepared for it and be ready to fight back.

Moving on to the next box, ask them to consider what OCD symptoms would be likely to come back and what would be the warning signs, for example they might notice more obsessions or feel more anxious. This should be again be framed as an important part of the plan, so they know what to expect OCD to do rather than be caught off guard. The next box is similar but asks what other people would notice if OCD returned; you can ask the parent to contribute to this box.

Moving on to a plan to manage this, ask the young person to write down who they would tell if they noticed OCD was coming back. Explain that they are not alone in fighting OCD and the reason someone from their family has been involved in treatment is so they have support outside the sessions. The rationale for telling someone is so they can think together about what to do. They are then asked to refer to their rules for challenging OCD to come up with a plan of what to do if symptoms come back. Ultimately, they should develop a hierarchy and engage in ERP tasks to tackle OCD. They are encouraged to tell someone and act early when they notice OCD coming back. Remind them of the OCD cycle and that, if they start doing things for OCD, the cycle will start to get stronger.

The final box gives the young person an opportunity to look back over what they have accomplished in treatment and think about what they are now able to do that they could not do when OCD was taking up their time. Explain that it is important to fill their daily lives with activities not related to OCD as it has a habit of trying to sneak in when people are bored.

REVIEW OCD

Administer the measure you completed at assessment in Sessions 7 and 14 and plot this on the graph in this section of the workbook. If the score has reduced, explore with the young person how they think this has happened. Listen out for anything they say that fits with the ERP model. Ask them to reflect on progress and set out what they still have to work on in the follow-up period, referring to the goals they set themselves.

PLANNING AHEAD

Remind them that they have to continue challenging OCD moving forwards. In this section of the workbook, they are asked to make a list of compulsions they need to work on before the next review session. They are reminded that they can download an OCD steps plan or timetable to plan this out. It is helpful for the young person to consider what they can do now that they could not do before, to reflect on how far they have come, and in light of this, you can ask them if they would like to add any more goals to their list.

CERTIFICATE

Share a celebratory certificate with them in their workbook to congratulate them on completing the weekly sessions and for all the effort they have put into challenging OCD.

Schedule in their review appointment.

APPENDIX

Things to Help You in Treatment

This section covers additional modules that can be weaved into treatment and includes:

- Different feelings
- Learning about thoughts
- Helpful thoughts
- Ask others to challenge OCD
- Do a survey or find out facts
- Managing ASD-related stress.

DIFFERENT FEELINGS

Often young people with ASD struggle to differentiate different emotional states, which can make identifying anxiety and measuring it difficult. In the Appendix in the workbook, they are given a list of different emotions and asked to think about each in turn, considering the physical sensations associated with them. They are invited to add additional examples for each emotion. The workbook summarizes the feelings of happiness, sadness and anger. The young person is also asked to consider other emotions that they experience. Throughout this exercise, you can ask them to think about how these emotions differ from anxiety. A useful homework task is to watch the Disney film *Inside Out* where there are characters to represent joy, sadness, fear, disgust and anger.

LEARNING ABOUT THOUGHTS

Some young people with ASD may not understand the concept of 'thoughts' and the different types of thoughts that we all experience. This may come up in treatment when talking about obsessions. Some young people with ASD may think they can get rid of intrusive thoughts or not have 'negative' thoughts and that CBT will help with this. They may benefit from some additional education, to build up their understanding of thoughts.

The Appendix in the workbook explains that everyone gets a range of different thoughts. We get unwanted intrusive thoughts that pop into our heads and we have deliberate thoughts we choose to have. It is important to share that intrusive thoughts can be scary, strange, horrible and rude, but they can also be neutral and pleasant. You can use their special interests to give some examples of positive thoughts that come into their head (they pop in and are not brought in deliberately). Examples of neutral intrusive thoughts can include thinking about what to have for lunch in the middle of a session. Intrusive thoughts are helpful for coming up with ideas and being creative, otherwise we would all be like robots. You can link this to their special interests; for example, 'If JK Rowling did not have thoughts outside her control, do you think she would have created the Harry Potter stories?'

Share the surveys that have been completed by Rachman and de Silva (1978) and Purdon and Clark (1993). The first study can be shared to give the message that everyone gets thoughts they do not like, and these are similar in young people with and without OCD. The important difference is that people with OCD get anxious about them, think they mean something and respond by doing compulsions. The second survey lists specific intrusive thoughts that were endorsed by university students without OCD. This survey is helpful as it lists a range of thoughts, including aggressive and sexual obsessions, which are very common for lots of young people.

You can encourage the young person to do a survey and ask you and their parent in session whether you get intrusive thoughts and what types. This is a helpful exercise as it enables parents to build insight into the fact that they too get similar thoughts, and this is part of normal human experience. It is important to share with the young person that thoughts are not facts, and particularly so with young people with ASD, as given their rigid black-and-white thinking style, they are more likely to believe that a thought that has popped into their head must be true. You can share some optical illusions to make the point that our brain can play tricks on us, but also, perception can change.

It is important to share that our brains come up with lots of thoughts all the time and most are random. We cannot control all our thoughts and we do not need lots of the thoughts we get. You can liken it to a spam filter on emails and that some emails will get through and we get lots of emails we do not need.

An exercise that might be helpful to share with young people who feel they should control or stop their intrusive thoughts is the 'pink elephant' exercise. You ask the young person (and their parent) to not think about a pink elephant in the corner of the room. Keep reminding them not to think of the pink elephant. Ask them to reflect on what happened when they tried to do this. They will discover that the thought of a pink elephant kept popping up. Some young people with ASD may not understand this exercise as they struggle with metacognitive skills to recognize what is happening with their thoughts. For those young people, a concrete representation of this can be more helpful – for example, throw a tennis ball against a wall to show that, the more you try to throw it away, it will just bounce back.

The purpose of the next section on learning about thoughts is to share how OCD can trick people to think our thoughts are powerful or can make things come true. To test this out, you can ask the young person and parent to do exercises set out in the Appendix of the workbook. First, ask the young person to think about something they would like to happen and something that is immediate, such as finding money under their chair. Ask them what happened and if it came true. Now ask them to think about something unpleasant happening, such as their parent getting hurt or cars outside crashing, again something immediate that can be tested out. Ask them to write down what they have learned about the power of thoughts by completing this exercise. It may be important for the young person to use this learning in their ERP tasks. This will allow you to link it more specifically to their own OCD symptoms. For example, an exposure might include thinking purposefully about a family member dying, or the young person vomiting after a contamination task. Can they make it come true just by thinking about it? What happens to their anxiety the longer that they think about it?

HELPFUL THOUGHTS

In the Appendix in the workbook, share with the young person that OCD can be like a bully and say lots of things in their head. Some people find it helpful to say something back to OCD to help them challenge it. It is important to ensure that what the young person takes from this is not to give themselves reassurance or say something to bring their anxiety down (a compulsion), but rather statements to encourage them to challenge OCD. They are given some options in the boxes or they can add their own. They may find it helpful to write these down and put them in places where OCD often gets triggered as an external reminder, such as by the bathroom sink or the front door.

ASK OTHERS TO CHALLENGE OCD

This should be a standard part of treatment, as we know (family) accommodation is significant and common in OCD. You can use this section to specifically think about tackling (family) accommodation along with the young person challenging rituals, or it could be an avenue to focus on if the young person is struggling to initiate or carry out tasks. Additionally, if you notice that families are struggling to identify what they or others are doing for OCD, you can use parts of this module to build insight and recognition into their role in the OCD cycle.

In the Appendix of the workbook, the module starts with normalizing (family) accommodation in OCD, so they do not feel blamed or criticized when completing this work. There are examples given of how OCD commonly gets other people involved, such as giving reassurance, helping with compulsions, avoiding things that OCD does not like and changing plans and routines because of OCD. Explain that all these things work in the same way as the young person's compulsions. They aim to bring anxiety down but actually work to keep OCD going in the long run. It is helpful to share that we know that parents are used to comforting their children to make them feel better – it is a natural and understandable thing to do. However, in the context of OCD, these parental reactions can serve to increase their child's anxiety over time. Given (family) accommodation is tackled in the same way as any other compulsion in OCD, they can use the ERP task sheets and hierarchies to help guide them on what to do. The additional thing to consider with (family) accommodation is that if more than one family member or people outside of the family – friends, teachers – are involved, it is important that everyone who is involved challenges OCD in a consistent way. This is especially important for someone who has ASD, so things are predictable and OCD does not sneak around to get what it wants.

In the workbook Appendix, there are some sheets to complete on reassurance seeking, as this can be difficult for families to tackle and they may need specific ideas on how to manage this. You will first ask the young person and parent to write down how OCD gets reassurance from others. This can include answering specific questions, saying certain things, asking their parent to eat something before they do to check it is not contaminated, or parents offering reassurance in subtle ways such as saying things will be okay, which they may see as a form of offering comfort, but OCD may see as reassurance. You then run through ideas with them to think about how to respond. It is important that the young person agrees to the plan and that they know exactly what will happen, again to make things predictable. Encourage the family to conduct the plan exactly as it is set out and not to change things over the week without discussing it further with the young person. They are reminded to ensure that everyone involved in accommodating OCD is responding in the same way.

DO A SURVEY OR FIND OUT FACTS

Surveys can be used in a variety of ways to support a young person with ERP tasks. Some young people have been doing their OCD compulsions for a long time, so they may have lost perspective on what is considered 'normal'. An added difficulty for young people with ASD is that they may be less receptive to noticing social norms as well as struggle to consider how others may think due to theory of mind difficulties (i.e. difficulties in the ability to attribute mental states – beliefs, intents, desires, emotions, knowledge, etc. – to oneself and to others). They may find it helpful to conduct a survey to find out the norm, so they have a sense of what they are working towards, for example how often do people go to the toilet, how much do they wipe themselves, how long do they spend in the toilet? Some young people may lack insight into the irrationality of their fear, for example they may believe all cheeses have worms in them. There is a page in Appendix of workbook called 'Do a survey or find out facts' to help young people set up a survey or find out facts.

Once the rationale for the survey has been set up, support the young person to carry out the survey by noting down what they will search for – what are the search terms, who will they ask, where will they search? – and then once they have completed the survey, to write the results down and reflect on their learning.

It is important to explain to the young person that the survey is something they only complete once on each topic. This is to ensure it does not become a compulsion, for example the young person telling themselves the results over and over or checking that the results were correct. Remind them that we will know something has become a compulsion if it brings their anxiety down. Surveys are something to help them move forward in the ERP tasks.

MANAGING ASD-RELATED STRESS

Young people with ASD often experience higher levels of baseline anxiety. This can sometimes make their ability to undertake ERP tasks or move up the hierarchy more challenging. It can be helpful to augment the treatment with some of the following additional tools to share with the family to help them manage ASD-related stress:

- Visual schedules for the day (including when to do CBT homework).
- Keeping structure and predictability during the day (where helpful). Supporting the young person to know what to expect ahead of time, for example showing them pictures, using social stories, showing videos of where they are going.
- Giving them time to calm down during the day, for example having a quiet time to relax when they get home from school.
- Minimizing sensory stimulation when they are feeling overwhelmed and doing things in small doses.
- Thinking with them about how they can schedule in exercise and sensory activities to help reduce stress levels.

Dr Tony Attwood (2004) has developed *The Emotional Toolbox* which details physical activity, social, thinking, special interest and other tools that can be used by people with ASD to manage anxiety. It is important these tools are used as part of the young person's daily routine and are not implemented in response to the high levels of anxiety associated with completing an ERP task. If this becomes the case, this can undermine the principles of ERP (that anxiety habituates without the need to do anything) and there is a risk the strategies can become ritualized and compulsive, hence feeding into the OCD cycle.

FOLLOW-UP 1–4

Review Progress and Plan

FOLLOW-UP 1-4

- Set agenda
- Review and plan
- Review and measure OCD
- Looking to the future (Follow-up 4)

SET AGENDA

As with all sessions, set an agenda at the beginning of the session. You will find the young person and parent may have more to add to the agenda when asked, given there has been a longer time between sessions. Ensure that you give yourself enough time to review and plan. Share with them that the focus will be on reviewing how things have been since the last session and planning ahead to the next follow-up.

You may find in the review session that completing an ERP task may be helpful; this may be due to the young person losing momentum with completing tasks or they may be struggling to think of a way to challenge a particular part of their OCD, so doing it in session might be more helpful than planning it.

REVIEW AND PLAN

Ask the young person to review the plan they set out in their last session and reflect on what went well and what may be been difficult to manage. Ask them to think specifically about what OCD symptoms they have kept away, and which ones have been challenging. Using the same materials as before, invite them to look at their relapse prevention plan in their workbook (Session 20) to review if they think that what was included is still helpful or if this needs to be changed. You then move on to planning how to tackle anything that has been tricky to manage or anything they are still working on using the relevant sections of their workbook. Ultimately, this comes down to them planning and doing regular ERP tasks. They are given an opportunity to think about any potential barriers to them following through the plan they have come up with and are encouraged to think about how to work around this.

REVIEW AND MEASURE OCD

As you have done in other review sessions during treatment, take a measure of their OCD using the same questionnaire or interview schedule you used throughout treatment and plot this on their graph. Taking a measure of OCD is optional at Follow-up 1, as if this takes place one month after the end of treatment, this may have not allowed enough time to detect change.

Ask them to reflect on progress and why they think they got the score they did. If they are disappointed, support them to think about the plan they have detailed with you in session and how this can help them move forward.

LOOKING TO THE FUTURE (FOLLOW-UP 4)

In their final review with you (Follow-up 4), ask them to look at the goals they set themselves during treatment and think about the ones they have achieved and which ones they have not yet managed. It is helpful for young people with ASD to have a concrete plan to move forward, so you can spend some of the session developing this with them. You want to give a hopeful message and ask them to think about what they are looking forward to in the future. It is important to emphasize that they know how to challenge OCD and they have learned everything they need to know, so they should not forget to use their workbook to help them in the future.

References

Attwood, T. (2004). *Exploring Feelings: Cognitive Behaviour Therapy to Manage Anxiety*. Arlington, TX: Future Horizons.

Elliott, S. J. & Fitzsimons, L. (2014). 'Modified CBT for treatment of OCD in a 7-year-old boy with ASD – A case report.' *Journal of Child and Adolescent Psychiatric Nursing*, 27(3), 156–159.

Farrell, J. L., James, C. S., Maddox, B. B., Griffiths, D. & White, S. (2016). 'Treatment of Comorbid Obsessive-Compulsive Disorder in Youth with ASD: The Case of Max.' In A. E. Storch & B. A. Lewin (eds), *Clinical Handbook of Obsessive-Compulsive and Related Disorders: A Case-Based Approach to Treating Pediatric and Adult Populations* (pp.337–355). Cham: Springer International Publishing.

Geller, D. A. & March, J. S. (2012). 'Practice parameters for the assessment and treatment of children and adolescents with obsessive-compulsive disorder.' *Journal of the American Academy of Child & Adolescent Psychiatry*, 51(1), 98–113.

Griffiths, D. L., Farrell, L. J., Waters, A. M. & White, S. W. (2017). 'Clinical correlates of obsessive compulsive disorder and comorbid autism spectrum disorder in youth.' *Journal of Obsessive-Compulsive and Related Disorders*, 14, 90–98.

Jassi, A.D., Fernández de la Cruz, L., Russell, A. & Krebs, G. (submitted) 'An evaluation of a new autism-adapted cognitive behaviour therapy manual for adolescents with obsessive-compulsive disorder.' *Child Psychiatry & Human Development*.

Krebs, G., Murray, K. & Jassi, A. (2016). 'Modified cognitive behavior therapy for severe, treatment-resistant obsessive-compulsive disorder in an adolescent with autism spectrum disorder.' *Journal of Clinical Psychology*, 72(11), 1162–1173.

Lehmkuhl, H. D., Storch, E. A., Bodfish, J. W. & Geffken, G. R. (2008). 'Brief report: Exposure and response prevention for obsessive compulsive disorder in a 12-year-old with autism.' *Journal of Autism and Developmental Disorders*, 38(5), 977–981.

March, J. S. & Mulle, K. (1998). *OCD in Children and Adolescents: A Cognitive-Behavioral Treatment Manual*. New York, NY: Guilford Press.

Murray, K., Jassi, A., Mataix-Cols, D., Barrow, F. & Krebs, G. (2015). 'Outcomes of cognitive behavior therapy for obsessive compulsive disorder in young people with and without autism spectrum disorders: A case controlled study.' *Psychiatry Research*, 228(1), 8–13.

Nadeau, J. M., Arnold, E. B., Storch, E. A. & Lewin, A. B. (2013). 'Family cognitive-behavioral treatment for a child with autism and comorbid obsessive compulsive disorder.' *Clinical Case Studies*, 13(1), 22–36.

National Institute for Health and Clinical Excellence (2005). *Obsessive-Compulsive Disorder: Core Interventions in the Treatment of Obsessive-Compulsive Disorder and Body Dysmorphic Disorder*. London: NICE.

Purdon, C. & Clark, D. A. (1993). 'Obsessive intrusive thoughts in nonclinical subjects. Part I. Content and relation with depressive, anxious and obsessional symptoms.' *Behaviour Research and Therapy*, 31(8), 713–720.

Rachman, S. & de Silva, P. (1978). 'Abnormal and normal obsessions.' *Behaviour Research and Therapy*, 16(4), 233–248.

Reaven, J. A. & Hepburn, S. (2003). 'Cognitive-behavioral treatment of obsessive-compulsive disorder in a child with Asperger Syndrome: A case report.' *Autism*, 7(2), 145–164.

Rooney, M., Alfano, C. A., Walsh, K. S. & Parr, A. F. (2011). 'Differential diagnosis and treatment of obsessive-compulsive, inattentive, and sleep symptoms in a 7-year-old with PDD-NOS.' *Clinical Case Studies*, 10(2), 133–146.

Russell, A. J., Jassi, A., Fullana, M. A., Mack, H. *et al.* (2013). 'Cognitive behavior therapy for comorbid obsessive-compulsive disorder in high-functioning autism spectrum disorders: A randomized controlled trial.' *Depression & Anxiety*, 30(8), 697–708.

Russell, A., Jassi, A. & Johnston, K. (2019). *OCD and Autism: A Clinician's Guide to Adapting CBT*. London: Jessica Kingsley Publishers.

Scahill, L., Riddle, M. A., McSwiggin-Hardin, M., Ort, S. I. *et al.* (1997). 'Children's Yale-Brown Obsessive Compulsive Scale: Reliability and validity.' *Journal of the American Academy of Child & Adolescent Psychiatry*, 36(6), 844–852.

Shafran, R., Frampton, I., Heyman, I., Reynolds, M., Teachman, B. & Rachman, S. (2003). 'The preliminary development of a new self-report measure for OCD in young people.' *Journal of Adolescence*, 26(1), 137–142.

Steensel, F. J. A., Bögels, S. M. & Perrin, S. (2011). 'Anxiety disorders in children and adolescents with autistic spectrum disorders: A meta-analysis.' *Clinical Child and Family Psychology Review*, 14(3), 302–317.

Turner, C., Krebs, G. & Volz, C. (2019). *OCD – Tools to Help Young People Fight Back! A CBT Manual for Therapists*. London: Jessica Kingsley Publishers.

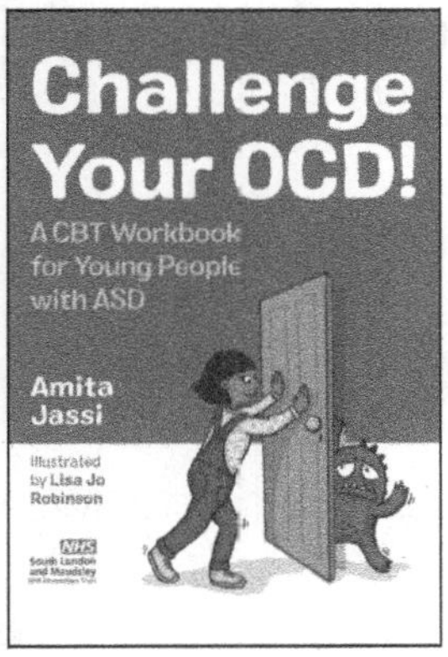

Challenge Your OCD!
A CBT Workbook for Young People with ASD
Amita Jassi

£19.99 | $27.95 | PB | 240PP | ISBN 978 1 78775 286 3 |
eISBN 978 1 78775 287 0

OCD is particularly prevalent in young people with ASD. This workbook, structured as a flexible 20-session programme, adapts CBT treatment to the specific needs of young people with OCD and ASD.

The workbook uses simple illustrations and diagrams to explain ways to challenge OCD thoughts and behaviours and includes fun and engaging activities for use within sessions and at home. An essential resource for clinicians treating young people with OCD and ASD, it will encourage and engage the young person in their recovery process.

This workbook is intended to be used in conjunction with the clinical manual for this title, Challenging OCD in Young People with ASD: A CBT Manual for Therapists.

Dr Amita Jassi is a Consultant Clinical Psychologist at the Specialist OCD, BDD and Related Disorders Clinic for young people at the Maudsley (UK), where she is lead clinician and researcher for those with OCD and ASD. She has been working with this client group since 2006 and teaches and trains clinicians in the treatment nationally and internationally.